T0104696

SPIRIT IN MOTION

GYM & WATER FITNESS / YOGA
BREATH-STRETCH TECHNIQUE

DR. WENDY GROSS

authorHOUSE®

AuthorHouse™
1663 Liberty Drive
Bloomington, IN 47403
www.authorhouse.com
Phone: 1 (800) 839-8640

© 2015 Dr. Wendy Gross. All rights reserved.
2nd Edition

Photographs and illustrations by Wendy Gross, EdD.

No part of this book may be reproduced, stored in a retrieval system, or transmitted by any means without the written permission of the author.

Published by AuthorHouse 11/23/2015

ISBN: 978-1-5049-5489-1 (sc)
ISBN: 978-1-5049-5488-4 (e)

Print information available on the last page.

Any people depicted in stock imagery provided by Thinkstock are models, and such images are being used for illustrative purposes only.
Certain stock imagery © Thinkstock.

This book is printed on acid-free paper.

Because of the dynamic nature of the Internet, any web addresses or links contained in this book may have changed since publication and may no longer be valid. The views expressed in this work are solely those of the author and do not necessarily reflect the views of the publisher, and the publisher hereby disclaims any responsibility for them.

The author and publisher of this book are not responsible in any manner whatsoever for any injury which may occur through reading or practicing the exercises in this book. Always consult a physician before beginning any exercise program as these activities may be too difficult and dangerous for some people. It is important to have a qualified instructor present and observing when practicing these exercises.

Wendy Gross, EdD
wlgross@earthlink.net

TABLE OF CONTENTS

INTRODUCTION

This book is about experience, your will, and sensation projected through space. Understanding the physical activity you perform allows your mind to guide your energy. You create movement which in turn re-creates your bodily home (personal bio-environment).

Upon reading this book, the novice at physical exercise may learn a meaningful approach to movement. The more experienced person will more fully grasp and benefit from this experience. When you use the techniques outlined in this book, you are learning to gather and direct your own energy. Breath-Stretch is the physiological event that is used to guide you. Relaxed attitude induced by Breath-Stretch can be used in all physical activities. However, all the reading accomplishes nothing until you feel a change in yourself.

This book is a guide to help you tap the energy source within yourself. You will learn to gather and release energy from the deepest recesses of your body and mind. Breath-Stretch creates new room for the tissues that comprise your body, enhancing circulation and allowing deep relaxation. Experience is a gift you give to yourself. Creative use and development of energy can benefit all aspects of your life.

I developed this work because in all my years of physical development (sports, dance, yoga, tai chi chuan, swimming), the understanding of what the instructor indicted when he or she mentioned force or energy remained unclear. It was as though the concept were spoken of or honored but not experience directly or not shared with outsiders.

Breath-Stretch and energy have never been explained simply, in such a way as to be made accessible. This text teaches how to produce a greater sense of well-being and how to re-create yourself through consciously directing will and desire. You can learn to experience freedom without bounds by directing energy to expand the deepest recesses of the body, mind and spirit.

If the Eastern masters are not available to us or are unwilling to share their secrets, than we will go directly to the source, the essence itself, and ask to be informed. The Eastern mysteries can be discovered by you. Have confidence and begin your own discovery!

Love feels exhilarating, comforting, and expansive. Breath-Stretch projects love. It sends the healing force generated by love, which is gathered from the life energy around you into your personal bio-environment.

In order to bring these new movement experiences to you in their fullness, this book explains the concept behind them; explores a few standard weight training exercises; and presents general postures and breathing techniques, which serve as a vocabulary of movement. Role of massage in healing is also considered. Most important, this book encourages you to evolve your own style of motion.

When incorporated into all motion, Breath-Stretch increases your movement potential. The breath expansion involved helps absorb the shock that motion produces. Although Breath-Stretch helps in shock absorption you must perform each movement carefully and in a manner that will not cause undue strain or pressure to the body.

Creative Breath-Stretch awakens and enlivens us. Best of all, it brings pleasure. The varied physical positions used with Breath-Stretch were developed to relax, stretch, and strengthen your whole body. Your body's inner movements massage the organs, glands and muscles. These techniques can be performed without strain or difficulty and are helpful when performed correctly. Once you begin to practice Breath-Stretch and adopt a Breath-Stretch approach to motion, you will begin to see and feel the effects of remolding your body and mind.

This book avoids excessive use of foreign languages, as they do nothing to help us reach the direct experience we need. The experience guides the changes which are subtle and dynamic. Personal experience removes doubt because this is not an intellectual practice. It is a feeling or sensation, not imagery. This work is presented in the hope that as you practice the techniques that you will find the sensory pathway easily.

Remember: Build up your vocabulary of sensation. Vocabulary is acquired by learning the physical feelings that the body experiences as it changes. Use sensual vocabulary to enable your mind to lead the energy through your body. Who is leading? The Spirit. A healthy person moves internally with grace and ease—in the dance of life. You are life. With each motion, you are creating yourself.

Guide yourself toward peace and joy.

CHAPTER ONE
Breath-Stretch

What is Breath-Stretch?

Breath-Stretch is a new non-invasive bodywork modality. This technique uses the breath and lymphatic sensations (physiological events) to project energy through space and produce a change in your mind and body. The energy surges are energy field movements, which can be channeled and directed. You can learn to gather and direct your own energy fields.

Breath-Stretch is the technique used to experience the essence of the Eastern meditation and movements arts. These arts stress the conscious experience and control of bio-energy or *chi*. Breath-Stretch uses the cardiovascular and lymphatic sensations as tools for developing a connection with the quiet yet profound forces within the body.

With Breath-Stretch you take one of the profound rhythms of the body – breath – and use its pumping action as it spreads throughout your being to activate each and every particle of yourself. This change is achieved through activating the senses and using concentration. The concentration itself changes the MOTION = MOVEMENT because the motion of thought can activate the energy system and change the internal environment. Breath-Stretch affects the "second circulatory system" (the lymphatic system) through pressure, which moves its fluids. Using conscious attention you can feel this motion of positive and negative forces and introduce yourself to force field subtleties. Here are two ways to understand the technique.

The Imagery Explanation

Splash! A stone is thrown into a lake. Ripples flow all the way to the shore even if we do not visually see the motion of the water at the shoreline. When you breath, the wave of inhalation extends outward into the space around you. The wave of exhalation releases you into a receptive atmosphere in which the force continues to move and project forward. Think of an archer. He or she draws the bowstring back gathering potential energy; this feeling is analogous to inhalation. When the string is released, kinetic energy is unleased as the arrow is driven forward toward its mark. Relaxation of contracted muscles which occurs in exhalation can be compared to the archer releasing the bowstring.

On the inhale phase of the breath cycle, potential energy is gathered. Envelope of the body is stretched with growing pressure. Upon the exhale phase of the breath cycle, pressure is released, allowing the flow of fluids while bio-electric energy continues its projected path through the body's energy field.

The Technical Explanation

Breath-Stretch is a natural, mechanical movement in which the body functions more efficiently. It is activated when the sensations of its motion are brought to conscious awareness. Mechanical effects of Breath-Stretch effect body systems. Most of us know that the role of the cardiovascular system is to circulate blood throughout the body with the heart as the pumping organ. Blood circulation is accomplished in a continuous, one-way circular flow. Lymphatic system is the body's other "circulatory system" with a few important differences. This system performs several important functions. It filters out disease-causing organisms; makes white blood cells and antibodies; and transports fluids, nutrients and wastes throughout the body as it drains off excess fluids and proteins left behind by the capillaries. Without the circulatory or lymphatic systems we would die. When either system is impaired we are debilitated.

The body depends on homeostatic (equilibrium-producing) mechanisms to maintain balance within all its systems. One mechanism that maintains the constancy of fluid in and around each cell in the body is the lymphatic system. Blood plasma from the cardiovascular system filters out of the capillaries into microscopic spaces between tissue cells due to the pumping action of the circulatory system. Most of the fluid is reabsorbed back into the blood the same way it exited. However, the non-reabsorbed fluid enters the lymphatic system. In the lymphatic system the fluid goes into a network of microscopic blind-end tubes (lymphatic capillaries) which drain into larger vessels (lymphatic venules and veins). Finally, fluid in the lymphatic system flows into terminal vessels called the right lymphatic vessel and thoracic duct which both empty into veins in the neck. The lymphatic fluids drain into dumping sites in the lower neck. The system can be thought of as the fluid run-off of a drainage system.

Remember: The lymphatic system has a one-way movement and does not flow over and over through a circulating system with a pump like the heart. The lymphatic system is moved by the pressure of breathing (by the diaphragm and external intercostal muscles), muscular movements and pressure from adjacent blood vessels.

Activating Breath-Stretch

The energy referred to in this book is *chi* or *prana*, which is universal energy (electromagnetic energy, heat, light). The universal energy localized within the body is called bio-electrical energy.

When the mind concentrates on any physical system the system listens, perks up. It is as if your name was called and you respond by opening up and becoming receptive to new information. As concentration on breathing deepens, expansion, release and surge motions can be felt throughout the body. Through meditation, you can become aware of the breath wave moving all the way out to the tips of the toes/fingers and to the top of the head.

To release specific tension blocks within the body, place the body in a passive, stretched position. You may stretch the neck laterally to the left or right. To activate Breath-Stretch bring the mind to the area experiencing tension by placing a hand over the area or stroking it to focus and activate sensual responses. Inhale slowly, feeling the total stretch throughout the body. Upon exhaling, feel the full body release while focusing your mind on the specific area that you are relaxing. Since thoughts are electrical in nature, your thoughts will direct the flow of energy to the area you are mentally focused upon.

As you inhale, a subtle motion of lymph moves out and energy is gathered. Wait until the need to exhale returns to you; now, exhale, sending out the energy and directing muscular effort. This sensory path is already present within you and functioning. You are "turning up the volume" by feeling and leading its power.

Energy force is not the breath but can be channeled and directed to move along with the breath. You piggy-back the energy onto the breath. Over time energy can be felt as a separate experience, more powerful than the breath itself. Inhale feels like a strengthening of all tissues with the gathered energy pressing down into the bones. The sensation is one of a gathering force, relaxed and waiting. Exhale feels like an invisible lightening moving instantaneously at the beginning of the exhale and continues throughout the exhale as a sensation of active forces.

Deep breathing is an extension of the normal cycle of breath. By concentration and practice, the capacity of internal breathing space is greatly increased. Also, through breath control, the amount of effort exerted in a particular area can be observed calmly. If you can breath assuredly, then your concentration can turn to the actual energy performance since your internal timing mechanism is slowed down.

When you use Breath-Stretch, energy is passing through your entire system. As you physically invite energy to live within you, the system opens. With time the capacity and experience grow. The internal organs are stretched and expanded in the physical exercises – not shocked or torn. Use Breath-Stretch to buffer internally and create a non-shocking, smooth, elongated flow of motion (energy). The health ramifications of motion are the massage and electrical charge/exchanges within your tissues.

Ecstasy of movement develops the physical body. The gym is an area for self-evolution: ecstasy, happiness, energy, and thrills. Before you move physically in space, imagine the movement and give off energy. As you move, realize that you are not limited by your body, the walls or the building. Your body disappears in the flow of motion.

Depending upon your genetics, age, and physical history, the body will exhibit your Vital Force (energy) in different ways. In all cases, the goal is to experience pure Vital Force. The thrill, peace, and freedom which this experience yields are well worth the journey.

You are the Vital Force. You are the conscious life force temporarily playing in matter. As matter you are limited by physical conditions, but the scope of the physical world and your bodily experience can be expanded through breathing and stretching the boundaries.

Strength and pleasure of pure magnetism that you experience allow you to feel your link to the universal energy. It is a full-body experience generated from the solar plexus and abdomen. Breath-Stretch speaks to the whole person - drawing the healing of loving sensations from the energy around you into your bodily home.

Breath-Stretch and Sensual Imagery

Use of creative imagery will enhance the effectiveness of Breath-Stretch and help you *feel* the experience. Close your eyes and as you inhale, imagine a hand moving out from the diaphragm area toward the area to be relaxed. The body has no shape when your eyes are closed - search the darkness for any discomfort. Localize the area in the darkness. Know where it is in space and concentrate on it. Now, travel toward the area along with the breath as the inhaled breath creates a pressure buildup and pushes outward. The exhale releases the pressure and sends the force to release the pain or block.

When you inhale, the swelling of the body pressing against the body's envelope (your skin) causing a pressure-pump that affects the entire body. Your body is similar to a balloon as your breath pushes outward from internal spaces. Pressure is most easily felt and activated close to the source of the motion. During this pressure phase, energy is gathered. As you exhale, you will feel the release of the pressure and the movement of fluids that flow gently forward within the lymphatic system. This release is NOT a relaxation in the sense of a collapse. Rather, the energy in your being is now projected or moved outward in space as a force.

Inhale all the way down to the center of your being and feel the pressure all the way out to the smallest area. The desire to reach further is the dynamic push that sends you deep inside, helping you gather the energy that carries a push of expansive force that buffers all the spaces within your tissue. Feeling as you inhale is one of air pressure wanting to continue to increase. The body would take in more air if possible. The throat is open and the space inside the body expands from the pressure that moves the skin outward.

Exhale allows you to release breath and send energy outward while transforming the body's physical position and allowing the body to establish a new norm or base position. Without this re-establishment of balance within your tissues between pushes or Breath-Stretch, the force would tear your joint or tissues at their weakest points.

Technique: Pinpoint

Always pinpoint the area to which you need to send the Breath-Stretch. Put your hand on the area or lean against an object and rub the surface to bring sensation to the area. Concentrate on the sensation of the breath motion as the area expands and releases. Welcome people observing you because their stage of physical and spiritual evolution will never correspond to yours. Your evolution invites others to explore.

Breath-Stretch and lymphatic movements are physiological events. Energy surges are field forces movements that can be channeled and lead. In this book you are learning to gather and focus your own energy. Center the mind in a relaxed body to gather energy and project it into space through the physical body.

Again, the energy force is not the breath but can be channeled and directed to ride along with the breath. You mentally attach the energy or *chi* onto the breath.

Remember: Inhale is like the gathering of forces before a lightning strike. The strike of lightening, before the eye can see it, is the energy-sending phase. You should imagine the sight and sound of lightning in the sky while you exhale and feel the experiences as if they were a great surge of energy --- like a lightning strike --- the effects linger after the strike is accomplished.

Use Breath-Stretch to expand your energy throughout the whole body and beyond the skin to earth, sky and horizons—every spot on the sphere that surrounds you. Feel the energy continuing to thrust out into space as the air exists the lungs. Energy moves instantaneously. The lymphatic system will follow the motion of the breath but move more slowly than the breath. At the beginning of the exhale the energy is sent out toward its mark and continues moving throughout the exhale phase and the period of waiting to inhale.

Why do physical education courses ignore breath expansion?

Western culture has a history of splitting the mind and body. The mind is elevated and the body debased. The mind-body split allowed us to treat the body as a machine. Care of our basic bio-energy or spirit has been overlooked. Our yearning for spirit in the culture at large is a response to this loss of contact – direct contact, direct experience - a feeling of connection with the natural wonders with which we are one. As we unite the mind and body with spirit, we create an atmosphere that prevents illness and helps maintain health. Eastern philosophies offer a profoundly different insight into life and the control of our physical evolution. These cultures have integrated breath and energy into the martial, meditative and healing arts. Principles of energy motion through positive and negative flow have long been passed from teacher to student. With the growing interest on the part of Western medical and physical arts, come Eastern techniques are being revealed. Integration of these concepts into our culture is increasing every day.

While the Western world has developed the finest emergency health care system in the world, our understanding of the everyday physical body's maintenance is rudimentary. We need the spiritual connection. Breath-Stretch develops the basic energy system, which is universal and accessible to all people.

The connection between universal energy and each of us can be experienced. Very few people who have experienced the Vital Force in motion enter the literary arena. A few masters teach, and their students are truly fortunate to have a living example. There are also the people who do experience the unity of Breath-Stretch and are practicing but do not feel the need to share this experience with the general public. Another group of practitioners are persons who read about the Vital Force, speak about it and even teach. Hearing or reading about the Vital Force in ancient literature on the healing, martial, and spiritual arts in not the same as first-hand experience. It may take a novice a few years to determine which teacher is teaching from experience.

Experience should be your goal. The strength and pleasure of the Breath-Stretch when it joins with energy flow is a "soul rush" (feeling of the motion of pure magnetism) generated from the link between the universal and each of us. It is a full-body experience flowing first from the abdomen. This is where the *dan tien* is located (an energy center approximately one- and one half inches below the navel and several inches within the body). There are three *dan tien* regions: upper, in the center of the head; middle, in the solar plexus; lower, below the navel. As you evolve, the center of the soul-rush moves to the center of the head---behind and a little above the brow line. This upper region is what is traditionally known in hatha yoga as the "Third Eve".

This experience evolves as you do. Time, practice and experience create a sensually perceived union of the universal essence and you.

CHAPTER TWO
Power Within

Sleeping Giant

During the 1960s and 70s our culture, experimented with altered states of consciousness produced by drugs. However, if you alter the physical state with drugs to induce a heightened awareness, you are deluding yourself. A person can become dependent on an artificial substance to gain entrance into a world, which is a gift that can be awakened by introducing oneself to deeper perceptions--- the sleeping giant within.

To use drugs because you feel that you are too rigid to experience the interior sensations without drugs is to take what appears to be the easy way out. In fact, it is ultimately the more difficult course. Drugs lead you to believe that the power of the drug itself takes precedence over the natural power within you. The tapping of the Vital Force within you liberates the psyche from dependence on outside assistance such as drugs, addictive relationships, and other crutches, while linking you with the life force.

To depend on mind-altering drugs is to become a slave to a lie: the belief that you are not complete, not whole. Accepting yourself with confidence sparks a light. The soul respond with delight.

We always live in a naturally drug-induced state, since we are matter that is composed of chemicals bonded together that continually change chemically to survive. Introduction of any substance into the body system such as food, water or air yields a change at the cellular level, which impacts the magnetic field within the body.

Thought, itself, changes the magnetic field and thereby altering an individual's state of being. Mind is constantly gathering information from all sources, originating thoughts, and remembering. Even intuitions (thoughts of unknown origin) are formed within the physical field through organic matter, which is altered by chemical shifts produced be the will (energy). The brain is the physical center of the mind. However, the mind's creative domain remains the magnetic force-field (ethereal body) in which thoughts form and mingle. Thoughts then motivate mater to become and change.

We are drugged by the thoughts we accept as true if we are no longer open to questioning or evolution. Freedom lies in experiencing the pure life force that runs through all creatures. In essence, life force is pure thought that precedes the accumulation of matter – the accumulation of thought in temporal form. In the play Our Town a character recites his address from a letter, and the last qualifier is "the mind of God." This is a wry tribute to the power from which the tragedy-comedy of our life arises. The world is created from the inside out. A quiet, powerful, waiting *yin* state takes shape on the physical plane because of a force-causing yang impact that is transformational and creative. Thought projection becomes physical formation.

Reflection upon a few ideas may assist you in opening up to the possibilities around you in daily experience. To adventure requires stepping off the known path of predictability in order to expand perception. This book is about experience. Experience created in drug-induced states will not produce the experience of confidence and joy that you can create through application and training.

The physical body may be capable of performing many of the physical feats described in this book. However, don't be misled. It is not the physical feats that are your goal. The physical is only a by-product of the activity. Body will exhibit the Vital Force in the flesh. But the goal, the supreme victory, is the experience of the pure Vital Force.

The Link

Link is the union of the physical and spiritual essence through sensation. The truth is a concrete sensation. You do not have to accept any new religion of cult of perfection because all matter, all God's creatures, are complete and perfect, regardless of whether or not our culture accepts the way any particular creature looks or acts. These judgments do not taint the pure essence that is eloquently expressed in all living things. The words beautiful and ugly are subjective judgments on an experience. The Breath-Stretch is done without the thought of judgment, progress or regression, positive or negative. It is pure experience without judgment only that will lead sensation thorough space in a way that transforms you.

Survival Takes Precedence

To experience something new it is necessary to give up the projected feeling or physical expectations of what is happening, of what the end result will feel like. When the body and mind become quiet, the rush of a force feels like a gushing, pulsing geyser. But if the physical is distracted by a state of rigidity (non-energy-flow) or the mind is filled with thoughts of conflict, then the sensors of the subtle life force must struggle to maintain the body's stability; therefore, in this case the force remains active but not under your conscious control or within your perception.

When the body/mind is concerned with survival, perception of the life force can be obliterated by necessity. Survival is the concern of any creature. If a fight or flight (sympathetic nervous system) response is called for, then for the uninitiated or untrained the subtler forces recede. The skilled user of energy draws this energy rush into the parasympathetic (relaxed, highly charged) atmosphere, which transforms the energy into a surge of thrills.

The life force speaks softly, for its power is great enough to disorientate your matter, your physical body. Do not look for the human fantasy of a Rambo-like contact. If the force were felt in all its power and magnificence, then you would be harmed physically or disorientated mentally by the experience. Allow yourself to feel the eternal flow of the river of breath that moves softly, penetrating, encircling, and cradling you.

Do not compare your experience to the experiences of other people in order to evaluate your progress. Rather, share your experiences as one traveler to another, knowing the journey will be unique to the individual even though experienced through a similar bodily vehicle. Your psychophysical path will be unique, as you are unique. Listen to the experience, and as you participate, allow the sensations simply to be. Do not direct; do not expect. Perceive, feel, and enjoy the unknown. If you know what to expect, there is not exploration. To experience anew, you must be willing to "take on all comers."

Energy in and of itself knows no good or evil. It is our wants and desires that define an event as good or bad – within a universe that is evolving by way of forces far beyond this plant's limits. Throughout time, when threatened we have realized our diminutive status – in the face of forces larger than all of us. We reorient ourselves by feeling the Link with this energy in our being – Link with the eternal in which we are eternal.

Biggest Trap

Your development is the only reward. Physical achievements are the sign-posts along your path of growth.

The genetic, environmental, and cultural propensities that make up this complex human being will limit to some extent the progress made in the psychophysical sphere (mind/body). However, the limits are only boundaries to venture beyond. Your will activated in the human body becomes a catalyst that creates a new activity at the cellular level and transforms tissue. This is the synergic reaction of the mind interacting with tissue and causing a new state in which matter is recreated.

Will or spirit ignites the mind, thereby defying matter and causing new boundaries to be set mentally and physically. All athletes activate this force when going beyond whatever limitations the genetic, environmental, and cultural realities have set.   Kirlian photography projects an image of energy fields. The viewer sees that the field forces in the body are whole and are influenced by the emotional (electric) and physical (material) events. Awareness gives you the power to affect your psychophysical environment.

Those of us with limited physical capabilities (physically challenged whether through accident, birth or disease) have the greatest challenge and the greatest potential reward. Understand that it is not the outward physical achievement that is sought, but the more lasting and fulfilling state of serenity within you that is the supreme goal. The outward signs of achievement are just that – superficial.

When the mind is distracted, concentration is poor. Concentration on the breath will immediately center you with a physical feeling and re-establish your presence in the moment. Now, use a positive or neutral thought, no a negative one, to initiate thought.

Mind Centering

Positive: I can do it.
Negative: This is silly; everyone is looking.
Breath-Stretch: Do it! Concentrate yourself and the Breath-Stretch expansion. Project energy. Release.

Technician vs Artist

There are technical performers that hit every movement correctly but do not lead you to experience their art as if it were the fabric of your being. The artistic performer lives in every motion of his or her work as though the creation were meant for this very moment in time. You are an artist.

Evolving by Using Your Physical Vocabulary

In demonstrations of Breath-Stretch in this book some hatha yoga body positions can be seen. The word yoga means yoke and refers to joining in communion with the self and the world by direct concentration. Yoga brings equilibrium to the body and mind. Hatha yoga is one of many yoga systems developed in India. It emphasizes physical and spiritual education.

Many of you may have done hatha yoga and may be familiar with its practices. Those of you who know nothing of yoga can just perform the Breath-Stretch, and the same principles will be activated with no clouding of experience through the use of Indian terms. Experience is the teacher. This experience is within your reach. You can understand through sensations the meaning of the words. Practice makes words superfluous.

Evil Eye

Words are vibrations of energy in the form of waves. Words are only the messenger, not the message. So, do not allow anyone to negatively influence your personal power (self-esteem) with words. Your own sense of wonder and will-power cannot be captured by anyone unless you allow it to happen.

The evil eye is an ancient term for the disturbance of one's energy field by another person. It is the capacity of another person to draw into and disorient the energy field of another person for his or her own purpose. Your way to safety is to center your feelings within the abdomen and lead your will to a greater power that draws you into the circle of cosmic energy and out of an individual's circle of power.

Concentrate on your own evolution. As your ability to concentrate increase, the ability to influence your own physiology will grow. During your practice of Breath-Stretch identify your own physical vocabulary of change that you can draw upon each time you practice.

CHAPTER THREE
Evolution

Principles Used in Physical Activities

The concept of Breath-Stretch movement is used in all three phases of physical development: static and dynamic body positions; breathing techniques, and meditation or prayer.

Breath-Stretch is a concept of movement that is utilized throughout the series of exercises developed and explained in this work. Once understood, the techniques can be used in all sporting activities and life situations.

All forms of education endeavor to create or evolve our beings (body, mind and spirit). All movement is an expression of our total personal experience at the moment when we are moving. This is what is missing in weight training. Weight training with soul or dance-like feeling will evoke a profound link with the energy fields. People lifting weights while concentrating the field force and direction prevents the inhibited movement so often seen in the weightlifters. Full strength is tapped by drawing on the forces of the universe, which your system is plugged into already then drawing and projecting the flow of energy through the body and outward into space. Like the cardiovascular system this is a full, continuing circle of energy that passes through us and the universe.

Breath-Stretch has its own timing. An adult breathes 12-18 times per minute. So the lymphatic system gets a pump from the breathing muscles which, when synchronized with the rhythmic motion of the weight movement, brings an individual into the realm of soul dance. Ordinary weight room workout is mechanical, lacking the heart and soul that lifts movement into the realm of dance/expression. Movement need not have the emotional element directly applied to the movement in order to be soul dance, but it must have rhythm and projection of will into space in order to be an evolving expression, a living bodily experience. Without the heart and soul the movement loses its life force. Also, the internal organs, joints and body systems are jammed up within their cavities, and this constriction strangles the flow of body processes. While the increased circulation of ordinary weight training temporarily feels good, the result for some individuals may be the increased potential for illness.

With Breath-Stretch, use as little weight as possible to maintain smooth, controlled energy flow during the movements. Weight-room exercised preformed with energy, direction and Breath-Stretch automatically propels an individual into the realm of dance, which is the force expressed physically.

If we have physical problem that the mind accepts as a permanent state, then the body will accept the truth of our own vision and protect (by avoiding or locking down) these areas, thereby limiting our bodily activities and movement possibilities. However, if we accept that the body is always evolving – just as maturing child has growing pains and physical discomforts – then the events are an invitation to develop ourselves in new ways. The physical body will accept this truth, and we can pass from one stage to another. Breath-Stretch is the link between the Vital Force and the physical body. This work is a guide to help you tap into this force within yourself.

As you travel through the adventure, your freedom of expression is only limited by the boundaries you set. Each spirit is evolving through the body. Certain permanent physical limitations are not to be denied, and should be assessed and understood. But Breath-Stretch can permit you to develop to the best of your physical ability. Spirit is the unseen moving will of the body – energy before it is projected. The mind is the caption. The body is capable of carrying energy. With a thoughtful approach the spirit leads the mind and propels energy through physical body bringing joy that is unbounded by time or space. Breath-Stretch is merely the training technique.

CHAPTER FOUR
Energy

Prana/Chi

Vital force can be felt in people as the bio-energy, a form of the universal *prana* or *chi*. The force transfers itself into the individual body, vibrating in waves that pass into and throughout the body. However, the individual can direct this same force within the body and change his or her force field by linking with the infinite. The Breath-Stretch, which moves in rhythmic motion through expansion and release.

Nonetheless, a person can use the sensation associated with Breath-Stretch to stimulate and open up a flow of energy by activating the will. Through a series of exercises, I will describe how to feel and project this Breath-Stretch, which will bring greater *prana/chi* to your being.

Language is a poor tool to describe that which is no ordinary physical event (but which, even so, lies within the scope of all creatures). The words I have chosen are meant to direct you toward sensation. So follow the instructions and then feel, feel, feel. What you sense will never exactly fit any description, but the practice brings an immense, sustained pleasure as you build a sensual rather than verbal vocabulary.

Realize as your body evolves that growth will entail levels of what can be described as discomfort. This is to be expected. You are re-creating your body from the deepest mental and physical levels. See yourself not as solid flesh and bones, but as a living force that has gathered and entered physical matter. You are spirit bring a body experience. Each molecule of your person is made of atoms which in turn can be split down to electrons, neutrons and protons, etc., that can be split further.

Quantum Understanding of the Body

The energy of the body is a force oscillating between positive and negative polarities.

Negative Polarity = *yin* in Chinese philosophy

Female, wave, slender, weak, listless, slow, gentle, pressure, with meridian flow

Positive Polarity = *yang* in Chinese philosophy

    Male, particle, well-made, strong, active, quick, strong, against-meridian flow

    The *yin* is passive, thought, cool waiting. It is just as important as the *yang*, which is active, forceful, hot, moving energy.

    To relax while in the *yang* motion means to project energy out along the line of the fascia (the thin strong tissue around muscled, etc.) while contracting the muscles to produce the movement. However, you must not strangle the muscles. Use about 80 percent of the effort to contract your muscle; then, lead the energy through the last 20 percent of space around the muscle. Open up the joints and organs in the 20 percent space and move energy through like light through a transparent tube. This is figurative description of a motion. If you lock down any areas while moving energy, it blocks your system and blows out or dis-eases the tissue, causing strain and illness.

    In each moment we create ourselves through consciousness. We are a gestalt (view) of consciousness. The body and mind are parts of one system. However, we tend to view the system in one aspect or the other --- usually the body because it seems concrete.

    Out of a waiting, pulsating energy source (*yin*), the physical (*yang*) is created. Upon conscious perception, a wave becomes a particle, the foundation of all matter. A wave being light, itself, momentarily poised as a particle becomes matter or suspended light. We pulsate in and out of the appearance of solid matter. From the mind, a swirling pool of pulsating energy, you create a will, a desire to be. If you choose to strengthen the force, then "will" the force to create the opportunity for evolution and development.

    Note in the following representation of the energy path that breath is the communication link between the mind and body. Breath-Stretch concentration strengthens the connection between the mind and body.

    Energy > Mind/Spirit > Brain/Body > World (Created)

Breath

    Modern physicists understand that matter is light momentarily collected or held in space/time by energy attractions. In actuality you are not a solid being. You are an energy wave becoming a particle through reflection. The element of consciousness makes all the difference. Consciousness with a purpose becomes a raison d'etre and a force to be reckoned with. Mind can direct this consciousness, and so form and change the internal physical body. Breath-Stretch allows you to project this energy by feeling the natural, subtle expansion/relaxation of tissue that is a manifestation of the force the consciousness can direct through the relaxed body.

Now, add the further realization that we are energy emanating from the source of all energy, and all parts can be traced back to the whole. We share a holistic experience of life/energy. The quiet, thoughtful, yin energy (wave) becomes active - physical, yang energy (particle), and we experience the patterns of particle interconnections that are a holographic image. Physical reality is an energy event in space. The power of your mind changes and develops this physical world. You are, on the physical plane, what you bring into being via thoughts on the mental/spiritual plane. To change allow the mind to perceive the physical experience anew without judging. We cannot see energy---only its manifestations. Some philosophers would say "God = Energy = Light."

Energy Descriptions

Western Vibration Field	Eastern View	Quantum
etheric (bioelectric)	*yin*	wave (electron level)
physical	*yang*	particle (living-cell level)
crystallized	world	things (human body)

The point of the above chart is that whatever you are, project and feel, is what you get. The body appears solid at this moment because at this particular frequency and form - this particular view point - matter takes on the appearance of solidity. Feeling of vastness, when evolved within the body, opens the area between molecules, cells, organs, joints, etc. allowing more motion between points in proximity. In Breath-Stretch, energy is gathered into these spaces before being directed trough them and released onto the physical plane. Your will or intention empowers the energy. This "meditation in motion" is quantum potential of the mind joining the plane of physical reality with energy. You make the wave into a particle and move the particle directly in space. You claim and empower yourself, recognize your energy, direct the force and move the particles of yourself. The energy becomes a "time hand" that can manipulate and move your cells, your whole being. Thought moves matter because it is light/energy in the form of molecules. Thought, being light, is energy that upon conscious direction can design or change matter (your physical being).

Your consciousness belongs to the unique individual that you are. Use this gift. The force will grow stronger and bring to you a personal understanding of the language of sensation.

Breath-Stretch in Meditation

All conscious thought creates energy which moves matter and impacts physical reality. Breath-Stretch done with feeling is a prayer that reaches out to meet the higher, greater forces with which we share the universe. You can feel the energy fields realign themselves inside the body field as the forces equalize and adjust with the universal fields.

Once the mind begins concentration, it leads energy through the body, and you are in a state of meditation. You are in a spiritual state. Prayer may or may not have words, but the sensation itself communicates and links you with the universal forces. Your will reaching out grows in strength as you use it. The opening and cleansing of the energy pathways will bring communication with the cosmic forces which will speak to you in a language of sensation. As you feel new experiences do not withdraw – rather, relax more deeply and observe. If you already know what to expect, then nothing new could happen. Feel. The experience itself will explain.

Where to Concentrate During
Moving and Static Meditations

As you begin to practice meditation in movement, place your focus on the spot one-and-one-half inches below the navel and about two inches deep to maintain balance in the physical exercises. This area is the lower *dan tien.*

If you do a static meditation, focus your concentration on the center of the forehead (Third Eye or Upper *Dan Tien*) and place your tongue against the roof of the mouth. This area is the upper *dan tien.* Your essence originated out of the pool of cosmic energy. Magnetic flows that are felt within your being are the pulls of positive (*yang*) and negative (*yin*) energy. When the flow becomes pure and full the experience takes on a cosmic connection so strong that it can be felt by the relaxed person who is conscious without judgment. The sensation is like the "heartbeat of the universe" which presses in upon you and flows through you, caressing the body like hugs; it thrills the body as the feeling passes around you, within you, through you.

To experience universal heartbeat changes the fabric of your being and brings into question all the ordinary values we live by. Experience bridges the gap between the seen and the unseen. You are liberated from the mundane. You are initiated. The world you live in is the same; yet, the world is experienced as wholly new.

Most texts emphasize the need for an instructor, but the soul will find its own way when the mind and heart are ready. Have faith in yourself. Know your limits but expand your horizons. Use common sense and the spirit of adventure to lead you own development. If a teacher appears, learn all you can but know that your path is unique. Enjoy your uniqueness. Would you want to live a life that is merely a copy of another's experience?

CHAPTER FIVE
Focus

The following exercises will allow you to learn to focus internally, deep within the body where movement originates. The attitude you feel is taken into movement, permitting a greater range of motion with ease. When motion begins from an awareness of deep relaxation and joy, steadiness, agility, endurance and vitality follow.

The exercises can be done alone or with another person. In either case after reading the description, assume the starting position. Suggest to yourself each method of internal focusing. Wait in quiet confidence for the experience to come to you, and the moment of ease and new sensations will appear. Everything you need to feel is present within you now. Expand your awareness through relaxed perception.

DEEP RELAXATION

Lie down on the couch, bed or floor – anywhere it is comfortable. Sit in a comfortable chair if you cannot lie down … Give all your weight back to the earth; allow the earth to support you – head, torso, arms, legs. The earth wants to hold you. Allow yourself to rest upon her, and she will lift you up.

Tense and relax each part of yourself: stretch out the right leg.; tensing the right leg, lift it a few inches and let it drop slowly to the floor. Roll the leg once or twice to insure total relaxation, and then forget about the leg. Follow this procedure with the left leg; right arm and left arm. Tense the buttocks, then relax; tense the abdomen by inhaling deeply and expanding the belly. Hold the breath to allow pressure to build. Open the mouth and exhale forcefully. Tense the upper chest by inhaling deeply – feeling the ribs open. Hold the breath; then exhale forcefully. Tense the shoulders by lifting them up and together in front of the chest with the elbows remaining on the earth; relax the shoulders. Tense and relax the neck by rolling from side to side. Squeeze the face together, pressing the tongue against the roof of the mouth behind the upper teeth; then relax. Stretch the face, open the eyes, stick out the tongue; then relax.

Go through the whole body with the mind, inwardly relaxing each part of the body following the sequence just described. Observe the breath as it slows without controlling the motion. The natural motion breath expands and relaxes with each cycle. Allow the breath to come to you and leave with its own timing.

As thoughts come, change and move on, observe the process without judging the thoughts. Feel the calmness behind the mind, a peace undisturbed by the mind. (If you fall asleep at this point, fine – that is what you needed most.) You are the stillness behind the mind and thoughts - a peacefulness that cannot be disturbed by the mind. You may return to this peace at any time, in any place, by returning to the breath. Remain quiet for at least 10 minutes.

Feel energy throughout your body and mind, radiating from the chest to all parts of your being and into the surrounding space above you, below you, around you. Breath will remain shallow, but the inhale and exhale will expand throughout the whole body from the tips of the fingers and toes to the top of the head. Allow the energy to the breath to be reflected in the chest as the breathing deepens. Allow the energy of the breath to be reflected in the fingers and toes as they begin to move with relaxation. Moving the hands and feet, then the arms and legs, take the feeling of restful ease with you. Stretch the limbs and torso, becoming fully awake. If you are lying on the floor, then roll over to the right side into the fetal position for a few minutes. Slowly come to a sitting position. Feel the effect of the deep relaxation.

After a few rounds of deep relaxation it is possible to reproduce the effect and benefit by going back to the sensation you felt through self-suggestion. You are creating a memory path through sensations. You can go back to the sensations. The feeling of total ease will reappear, whether you are driving your car, working at the office, dancing or resting.

Space Travel

To perform this exercise you should be either sitting or lying in a comfortable position. Close your eyes. Notice the light spots within the darkness of the closed eyes; watch the shape and color of these light areas change. Your eyes will become totally relaxed and receptive. Without fear, accept the darkness. You are in a sphere of moving particles in space. Inhale gathering force; exhale, allowing yourself to travel into the darkness by inviting it. Imagine you are in a spaceship heading out on an exciting adventure beyond the stars (the light points in darkness). The inhale brings the spots of light toward you, and with the exhale, you travel into the known. Wait, feel, experience and enjoy.

SELECTIVE CONCENTRATION: CREATING A MEMORY PATH

To perform this exercise you should be either sitting or lying comfortably. Select a part of the body, a portion as large as an arm or as small as a toe, or any organ or gland. Do not concentrate on the heart. Rather, focus on the breathing that affects rhythm of the heart. Bring your total awareness to that part. Feel the texture of the skin, the pulsation of the blood, the electricity passing through the nerves and the wave of lymph flow. Feel total alive in this area of the body. If you wish to move your hand, it moves. If you wish to feel the aliveness of the hand, feel. This can be done with any part of the body. Each area will relax; therefore, come closer to normal functioning.

You are creating a memory path, which you can travel along at any time in any place just by concentrating on the breath and sensations you have felt while doing this or any of the exercises in this work. Through the breath you can instantaneously travel back to the origin of the experience, and create the corresponding physical environment within your being.

Listening

To perform this exercise, you should be sitting or lying comfortably in a quiet room. Listen to the inward sounds. All the internal motions of life have sounds: high and low pitches, long and short pulsations or beats, rhythms of health or disease. Travel in the darkness to a place inward, particularly a place that is annoying because of pain. Listen with total interest. There is a message awaiting – you – a message spoken in the language of sensation. Send your own message to the area through Breath-Stretch. Hear the sounds as the breath slows. The body will reach total relaxation. You will be in a completely floating sphere with only sensations to guide you. Conduct your internal orchestra by suggesting that the sounds quiet down. Soothing and calming rhythms will be felt. Suggest by watching the breath and feeling the expansion and release of the Breath-Stretch as you witness energy and matter molding within you.

Man is in a state of total sound or vibration. You can perform the listening meditation while standing, sitting, or lying anywhere. Hear the sounds from the world around you: their texture, quality and rhythm. Feel the vibration of object such as cars passing, doors closing, people talking, music playing. Sound around us vibrates our flesh and bones: your own voice, the sounds you produce in your body, impact the body and create an atmosphere in which each cell vibrates. We cannot change the whole world around us. We can change its effect upon us and know that our own actions create the internal environment through which we perceive the outside world. We create our sensory veil.

Body Breath

Sitting or lying in a quiet place, bring your total attention to the abdomen. Feel the expansion and relaxation of the area with each breath, slowly in and out, in and out. Allow yourself to rest into the breath, slowing as the perception of total body expansion begins. Just as a wave of water ripples to the edge of the shore, so the wave-like motion of the breath moves throughout our body with each inhalation and exhalation. This motion is important. Motion is an essential key to deep internal relaxation. Wave-like motion and rhythm massages and enlivens every atom. The wave of breath is extremely subtle. However, with diligent practice you will experience this motion.

Indian philosophy speaks of *prana* or the vital breath of life. *Prana* is what you are feeling. You will begin to notice that it does not correspond exactly to the breath. But within the motion of the body it can be located as a field force moving around and through you, often pulsing forward and backward, in positive-negative, *yang-yin* waves or motion.

Surrendering: A Two-Partner Exercise

Have a partner sit cross-legged on the floor as you lie face up with the top of your head turned toward his or her legs. You should be flat on the floor with a small pillow under your knees.

Directions for the Lying Partner Exercise:

Relax completely. The sitting partner places his or her hands around your head, under the skull with the fingers slightly pointing downward, touching your neck. Lift your head directly up toward the ceiling an inch or two without lilting your head. Your chin and forehead should be on the same level. Surrender all your tension into your partner's hands. Give yourself completely. Feel the length of your neck as it stretches out from the head and down the back. Let yourself go. Relax into the darkness.

Directions for the Sitting Partner:

Your partner's elbows should be popped on your crossed legs. (The head is very heavy, over 15 pounds for an adult. That is why the weight of the head is used to elongate and release internal contraction in gravity-stretch positions.) You should wait to see if the person on the ground is or is not relaxed. Invite him or her with soft words to give the head's weight into your hands. Feel the pulsations passing between the head and your head's weight into your hands. Feel the pulsations passing between the head and your hands. You can feel the expansion of breathing move into and out of the head and skull.

Returning to the Lying Partner:

As a sensation the head, on inhalation feels like a balloon filling with water. You can feel this sensation through the skin, your head, and deep inside your body. On exhalation, feel as if the head is emptying out of the water and this release is a projection felt as energy being sent out of the body toward an external target, or into the body toward an area that is to be changed or healed.

Back to the Sitting Partner:

Before resting your partner's head carefully on the earth, pull the head gently toward you. Then slowly bring the head down. Leave your hands in position for a minute; then draw them away.

Final Step – Lying Partner:

Lie on the earth continuing to sense the after-effects. Slowly roll over to the side and sit up.

Deep Breathing for Relaxation: Three Parts

This exercise may be done while sitting in a chair or lying on the floor. It is a three-part exercise.

Phase One

Inhale, from the earth into the abdomen and feel yourself extend like a balloon into the space around you. Exhale and feel the abdomen flatten while the motion continues down to the center of the earth. Repeat.

Phase Two

Inhale, drawing the motion from the center of the earth into the abdomen. Now, deepen the inhalation so the mid-chest is extended into the space all around the body. Exhale, emptying the mid-chest and abdomen, following through back into the earth. Repeat several times.

Phase Three

Inhale from the center of the earth into the abdomen, mid-chest and upper chest. Do not raise the shoulders or tense the neck excessively. Float into the sky and wait for the need to inhale. Exhale, beginning with the upper chest (from the sky); then form the mid-chest; and finally, from the abdomen (into the earth). Repeat.

As the breathing in Phase Tree begins to come with ease, extend the uppermost point of inhalation and exhalation. Inhalation will float without tension up into the sky and will return to you. Exhalation will pass without tension down into the earth and return to you. At this point you will be learning to elongate the internal rhythms, the breath. So, do not "do" the breathing exercise. Rather allow the breath to float away up and come back to you on its own. Allow the breath to pass down and return to you.

Most important part of the exercise is the floating into the sky at maximum inhalation (which should be about 80 percent of lung capacity, as 100 percent would cause too much tension with the chest) and pause as you rest back into the earth at the end of the exhale cycle. The body will be in a state of neutrality, totally satisfied, and content. Body will have disappeared, and at the float-and-rest stage of the breath cycle, the breath also will have disappeared. What remains will be the *yin* force the quiet, waiting pool of potential energy that motivates the active *yang* cycle.

It is at the floating-and-resting stage that the body does not need to produce the larger activities involved in breathing and that the subtle forces of energy slip forward and take precedence. This is the most important moment for the beginning student to perceive the energy-field motion. The experienced individual can perceive these energy-field motions during daily activities and meditations.

Meditation Breathing for Opening Mind Centers: Yoga/Buddhist Method

Begin using the deep breathing sequence just described, and add a gentle lift of the genitals and anus during the exhale cycle. Gently press the tip of the tongue toward the roof of the mouth throughout the meditation. These added techniques close circuits of energy, allowing energy to flow around the spine. This flow targets the Third Eye or upper *dan tien*.

First, think of the inhalation as starting from the peritoneum (area between the genitals and the anus) and continuing up the spine to the area of the Third Eye or upper *dan tien*. Exhale down the front of the body, pressing the abdomen inward slightly to push out the air, and lifting the genitals and the anus slightly. Remember to float the breath into the sky and extend the breath down into the earth during the cycle. Practice a few cycles and over time increase the number of cycles. Relax into the quiet perception of the physical sensation created throughout the body by this exercise. The energy circuit will continue to flow without your conscious intention. Advance students can evoke this motion through thought alone.

The body naturally performs Buddhist breathing during a yawn. Observe yourself next time this physical event travels throughout the body. Breath is deep throughout chest and whole body; the ears close from internal pressure; and the abdomen contracts to increase pressure before the release of pressure that comes with exhalation. A feeling of contentment and restfulness follows.

DEEP BREATHING

Quiet Meditation (Buddhist)

INHALE
Release abdomen, genitals and anus
Inhale up through spine – mind follows motion to Third Eye

EXHALE
Slightly raise genitals and anus
Move abdomen in slightly
Exhale down the front of the body – mind follows motion

Movement & Weight Training Meditation (Taoist)

INHALE
Slightly raise anus and genitals
Slightly pull in abdomen
Inhale up through the spine – mind follows motion to Third Eye

Exhale
Release genital & anus
Press down through the abdomen and release
Exhale down at abdomen – mind follows motion

Targeting Area

To release specific tension blocks within the body, place the body in a passive position with gravity helping to stretch or elongate the body. Using Breath-Stretch bring the mind to the area by placing a hand over the area or stroking it to focus and activate sensual responses. As you inhale slowly, feel the total stretch throughout the body. Upon your exhale, feel the full-body release while focusing on the specific area, sending energy to it through the mind's projection of the force. Since thoughts are electrical in nature, the thoughts will direct the flow of energy to the area. (See Figure 1) Remember

*   Take long, slow breaths. The exhalation should take longer than the inhalation.
*   If the lower torso and hips are being focused on, use concentrated abdominal breaths; so, the expansion and release are localized.
*   If the neck, should and chest are being worked, use concentrated abdominal breaths, expand the release up through the upper torso and head.
*   If the arms or legs are being focused on, use the fingertips or ends of the toes to expand and exhale through.

DIRECT ENERGY OUT AT THE BEGINNING OF THE EXHALE

TO RELEASE TENSION FROM THE PROBLEM AREA

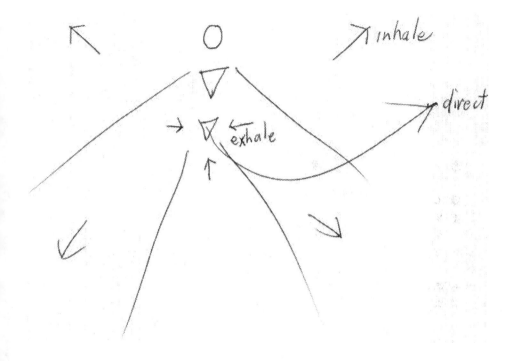

INHALE - expand breath
EXHALE - release breath
DIRECT - lead energy

CHAPTER SIX
Techniques

How to Approach the Exercises

An exercise is any position maintained with proper attitude. The external form can remain passive or active; the experience centers on the relaxed performance of particular muscular areas and the stimulation of glands and organs. Positions focus on blocks or constructions which are released from with the body through concentration and Breath-Stretch expansion.

Exercises Are Active and Passive

Care must be taken to practice these exercises correctly. All the movements have specific anatomical reasons be being performed. You are realigning, reapportioning, and revitalizing your whole being.

Active positions exhibit calm firmness – never a gripping that produces extreme shaking. You can never be totally relaxed while moving. So, contracting muscles to attain physical positions, you are using directed energy; the body is moving through space.

Example

Take your hand and make a calm, firm fist. Open you hand, and look at the color. Now, make a fist so hard that the hand begins to tremble. Open your hand and notice how white the hand is. It takes time for the proper color to return. Do not strangle yourself, your body, as you move. Rather, do slightly less than you are capable of doing. Do not compete, not even with yourself. Do not judge. Experience, feel, enjoy.

Passive positions are gravity-stretched. The body's weight is placed in the direction gravity is stretching or pulling the body. The body is not performing locomotion. It is moving through space passively.

Example

Hold your arm high over your head. Drop the arm, allowing it to fall freely toward the earth. This movement is the sensation of passive positions. Do an inner check to ensure that you are not tensing your head, shoulders, or other parts of your body. Your whole body should be relaxed.

Standing Tall

This technique is used to help elongate the skeleton-muscular system. We live with gravity always compressing and shortening joint spaces. Combat the pressure by visualizing the centrifugal and centripetal forces pulling on the body.

Imagine that the two forces want you. Feel the sky calling you up into him/herself as the centrifugal force of earth moves out and away from the earth's center. Feel the earth calling you down into herself as the centripetal force of earth pulls you down an in, toward the earth's center.

SKY (*yang*) Centrifugal force
EARTH (*yin*) Centripetal force

Yang is the bright, strong force of the sky. *Yin* is the dark, yielding force of the earth. The blending of *yang* and *yin* in harmony is health at its fullest. The body expresses these qualities through its health and motion. Just as the trees and branches are called up into the sky and the roots drawn into the earth by forces unseen by the eye, we give ourselves back to the forces of life once established in a position.

Energy + Direction

In physical exercise as in everyday activities, use and direct only enough energy to succeed at a task. We waste energy every day through unnecessary tension. A certain amount of tension is with us at all times. The heart beats, contraction to release to contraction, tension to relaxation to tension. However, using muscles groups not needed to produce an activity and overexerting the necessary muscle groups account for much of the lack of ease in everyday life.

The area most abused through hate, suspicion, lust, and greed is the heart. The mind becomes distraught or anxious when its wishes - often its illusions - are unfulfilled. And because the mind is always creating new goals, it remains in a state of uncertainty (tension), not enjoying the release or the relaxation needed. The heart is called upon to run after or harden against realities of life. For better health, practice Deep Relaxation (See chapter 5).

How to Breathe on Land and in Water

On land forward-bending exercises are begun with an exhalation: you exhale while moving into the position. Breathe normally while holding your body position; inhale when coming out of position. With practice you will begin to lengthen the inhalation and increase the depth of the exhalation. This will increase your breath capacity, massage internal organs through breath pressure and send a message to your physical being that all is well.

In water exercises inhale just before the head enters the water and exhale forcefully as you perform the underwater portion of the movement. All the air should already be expelled when the head exits the water. This will keep water from backing up into the nose.

Rocking

At all times use only enough muscular effort to perform a particular exercise. Allow the motion to slightly, gently rock you as it will. In water the rocking and water pressure against you will further assist the lymphatic system in moving interstitial fluid. On land the body will gently rock of its own accord in some movements. Notice the natural rocking and allow it to loosen up the areas that are directly affected.

Rocking is a fundamental form of motion that creates a soothing feeling, which is generated by pulsation. A pulsing motion mimics the push/pull, positive/negative, expansion/release activities or the energy force in *yang/yin* exercises. Each rotation is a push/pull of equal importance.

Rocking in all activities (rocking a baby) creates a sense of comfort naturally. Breath, itself, radiating throughout the body system creates a rocking rhythm, similar to waves in water. At certain points during exercises, use a gentle rocking to communicate security and blend your *yin* and *yang*. If you take command, then evoke the *yin* and *yang* in all your actions. The ensuing calmness in action, even in the most physically aggressive motion, brings you to a state the East has called "like a moon," a stillness where all motion begins.

The moon remains suspended above the earth by a balance of the centripetal (inward/*yin*) and centrifugal (outward/*yang*) forces of the cosmos. We balance the motion of the energy in our bodies by feeling both forces and allowing them to become balanced. Balance is not a static state but rather a position constantly being attained through the motion of forces adjusting.

Physiologist can relate balancing to the proprioceptors in the nervous system that upon stimulation sense location in space and delight in the push/pull sensation by releasing tension in the area related to rocking.

Injury

Recovery plans should become a part of everyday workouts. Our complex body will send messages you need to perceive and act upon. Messages tell you which areas are healthy, weak or show signs of strain. The body is constantly adjusting and compensating for injuries. Learn to identify a real sign of potential injury (weakness, pain, tingling) before a weakness becomes an injury.

As you think the body reacts. If you have a past injury that you think needs to be protected then the body will not allow you to develop the area to its highest potential. The body will shut down the area to protest it (called guarding). To evolve an area of the body that was injured in the past, realize very moment that you are changing and renewing.

At this moment - now – know you are recreating; yourself with each breath, each motion. Limited discomfort as you work out is the growing pain of evolution as the body changes. Learn to listen. Work within your range of growth – but no not overwork. You can limit your "rebirth" by clinging to the past. So, to be reborn new feelings and sensations are to be expected and enjoyed.

CAUTION

Before practicing any of the exercises in this book, consult your physician concerning your overall health and ability to perform these exercises.

Remember: not all of the exercises are within your skill level. Start slowly and cautiously. Do less rather than more. The body will easily perform that which it is prepared to do. If it hurts, stop!

Slight discomfort is to be expected because as the physical body changes, the sensations of heat and tingling are produced. However, you must listen to the signals produced by the body to distinguish the changes that are positive from those that indicate too much exertion or strain. Experience is the teacher, and you must evaluate the sensations to determine whether to stop or continue.

*When exercising in water, there is the added risk of drowning. Anyone doing water exercises needs to have someone **present** and **watching** at all times whether the person is a beginner or an expert.*

The author is not responsible for any injury to anyone. The ideas, procedures and suggestions contained in this work are not intended as a substitute for consulting with your physician. All matters regarding your health require medical supervision.

CHAPTER SEVEN
Weight Training

All exercises must meet an individual's physical needs. Do the exercises according to your ability and growth possibilities. The method explained here is internal and has the intention of developing and directing energy. But your understanding of the body position and proper alignment is also important. Consult a professional trainer if you need advice on positioning for each exercise.

Sequence of Movement Creation

1. Center the mind: calm, directed. Focus: understand the exercise.
2. Center the body, the lower abdomen, extending far into the sky and deep into the earth; form the decision to send energy.
3. Body motion: the first phase is a coordinated inhalation (storing energy, the negative motion), and the second is the energy sending exhalation (releasing energy, the positive motion).

First, do the exercise without any weights (mind focus). Next, do the exercise with light weights (mind focus and physical projection). Over time, increase the weight if you wish to gain strength.

Many books are available on the topic of standard weight room exercises --- names, muscles used, the sequence and frequency of training. I have selected only a few to demonstrate the energy-motion technique. Always extend movement from the energy center in the abdomen called the lower *dan tien* which is approximately one-and-one half inches below the navel. This is the physical home of energy, grounding center. There are two other *dan tien* centers in Chinese philosophy – at the solar plexus (middle *dan tien*) and the center of the forehead (upper *dan tien*). The upper *dan tien* is called the ("Third Eye") in hatha yoga. We are concerned with physical energy in this text, but all movement is spiritual in nature. Nonetheless, when doing exercises, it is helpful to be grounded as the body moves. So, use the lower *dan tien* as the center of gravity in movement. An advanced practitioner can extend from the upper *dan tien*.

Sequence of Movement Execution

First:	Spirit moves mind
Second:	Breath-Stretch
Third:	Breath causing gentle movements

Before Each Exercise

1. Position yourself as if to begin exercise. Do a body check. Sweep through the body from the toes to the head. Locate where you are weak, where you are strong.
2. Ask yourself where to contract and what areas to relax.
3. Mentally go through the exercise, performing it without injury.
4. Ask yourself how to breath during motion – when to inhale or exhale.
5. Look around the immediate area for people walking by and novices who may interrupt you.
6. Mentally perform Breath-Stretch using the full body for one cycle and relying on the lower *dan tien* to center yourself. On the second inhale, integrate movement with breath.

During Execution of Motion

1. Feel the muscle contraction and the bones sliding at the joints. Give breath to the joint spaces by opening the spaces, not by grinding the joints. Permit the Breath-Stretch to fill the body spaces when you inhale, buffering the joints and bringing nourishing energy. When you exhale, feel the release of the contacted tissues as energy is sent out through space in the direction the mind has projected.
2. Move the light weight slowly, in a relaxed manner.
3. Each of the following pages exemplifies movement exercises traditional in the weight room with some advanced innovations.

Recovery from Exercise

1. Check your body for areas that need to be stretched out after being contracted during the exercises.
2. Rest an appropriate amount of time considering the intensity of the exercise and the length of time taken in its execution.

Beginning preparation and recovery phase are just as important as the exercise. The mind leads the energy that moves the body. Conscious thought before and after movement are essential to healthy development.

Physical Breathing Method During Movement Cycle: Taoist Method

Using Deep Breathing as previously mentioned. However, the contraction phase is reversed, so read the instructions and follow them carefully. The Taoist method of breathing was developed primarily for aggressive sports and martial arts. This style of breathing is more appropriate for the development of external muscle and secondarily, internal strength.

The inhalation

1. Slightly tighten the abdomen while inhaling. Think of this as the protective sheathe for the organs in the torso that permits a greater store of energy deep within the abdomen that can be projected during the downward thrust at the moment of exhalation.
2. Gently lift the genitals and anus.
3. Inhale about 80 percent of your lung capacity, so that there is still room to move the body with breath pressure growing in the torso.
4. Release genitals and anus area as you begin to exhale.

The exhalation

1. Press down in the abdomen as energy is directed out of the body through the limbs and head. This press will also stabilize the internal body and prevent a shock wave from passing through it.
2. With the force driven downward through the legs, an equal force is driven out through the arms and head.
3. Use about 80 percent of the energy projection through the body so that the body can recover if another motion or force is needed for stabilization.
4. Muscle use should be light. Over time, build weight slowly. Internal energy will grow as external strength evolves.

This style of motion protects the vital organs, yet permits mobility of energy. It is important to also practice Yoga/Buddhist relaxed breathing because of the gentle massage it gives to the internal body. The Taoist style alone would be too hard and disruptive.

When you have completed a workout of about 30-45 minutes in length, sit quietly and commence relaxed breathing (Buddhist Method). This will help cool the body down and stabilize it. Remember: the principle remains the same throughout the exercises - use light weights.

During a series of repeated exercise, inhale on return to your starting position (negative motion) and exhale on exertion into the exercise (positive motion).

Another way of stating the above is the following formula:

Think

Lead --- Energize --- Action in Space

Feel

If you become confused, as to when to inhale and exhale, then experiment. The exhalation will usually be the motion that requires the most dynamic and dramatic expression of energy. But when experimenting with a new motion or whenever else you feel the need, then protect your joints and inner organs by inhaling during execution to increase the space inside your tissues and cushion any impact; exhale out of the motion. However, upon becoming comfortable with the movement sequence, you may return to the standard inhale-prepare/exhale-execute to achieve deep stretch and strengthening. When the body is inverted or slanted to begin an exercise, do not change the direction of the ground in regard to the breathing. The concentration throughout the breath sequence and motion remains the same. The following pictures demonstrate some weight room exercises. (Figure 2)

CYCLE OF MOVEMENT & BREATH

PREPATATION/RECOVERY PHASE
Energy – build internally
Breath – inhale
Attitude – return to beginning position (*yin*)
EXECUTION PHASE
Energy – send through movement
Breath – exhale
Attitude – exertion (*yang*)

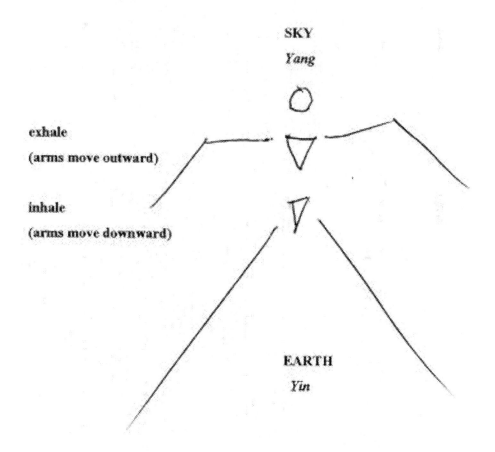

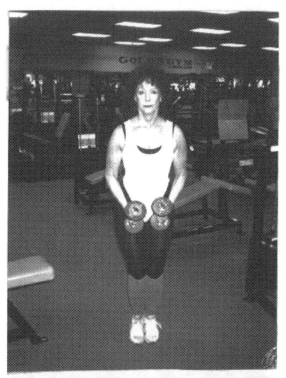

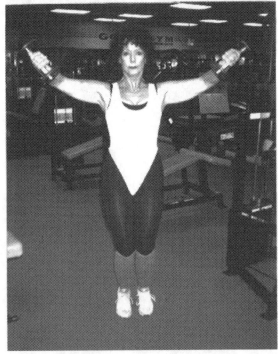

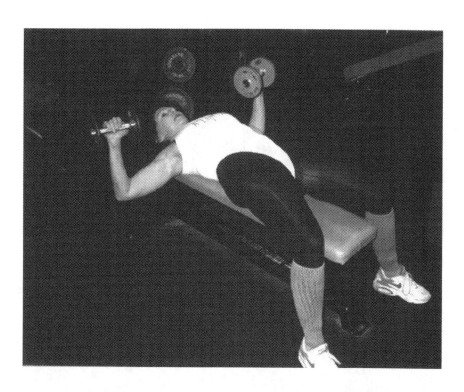

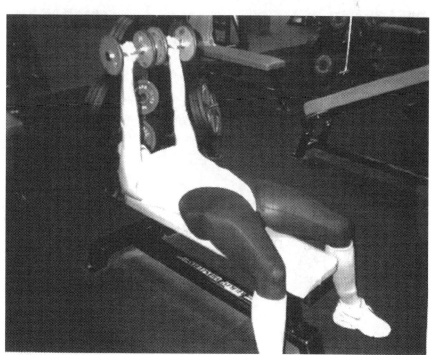

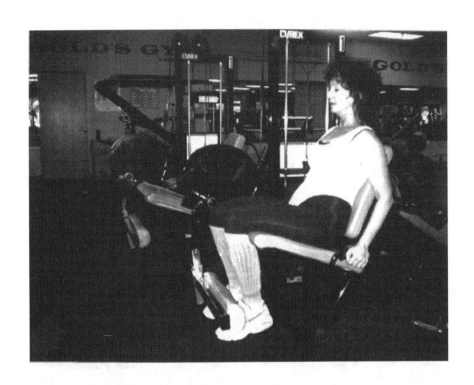

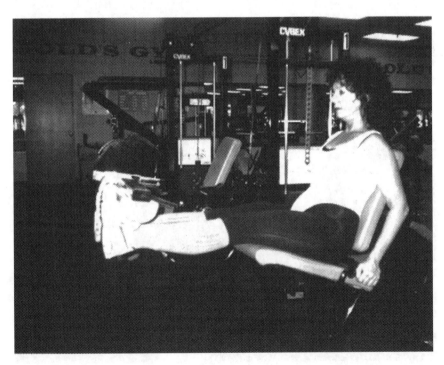

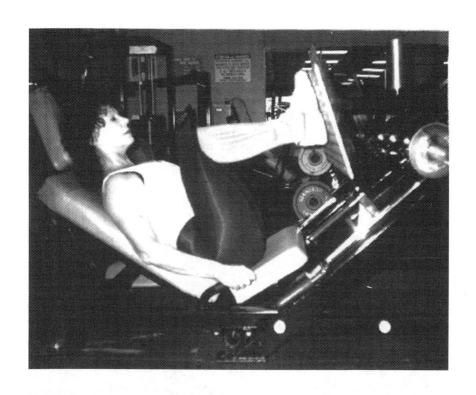

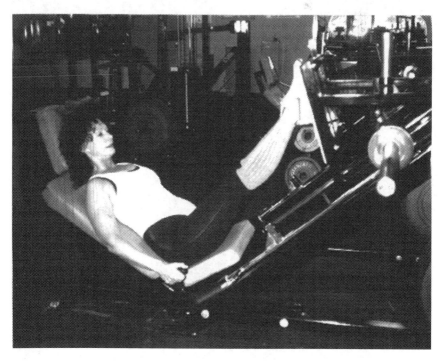

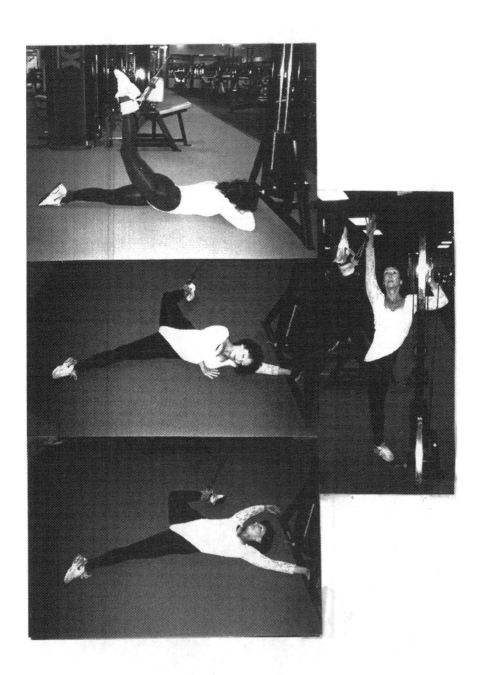

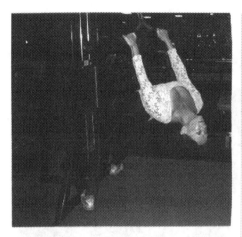

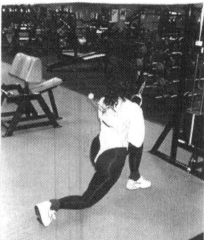

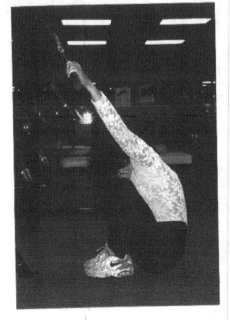

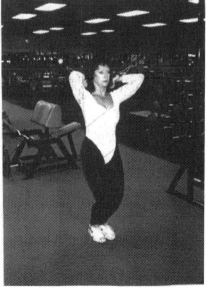

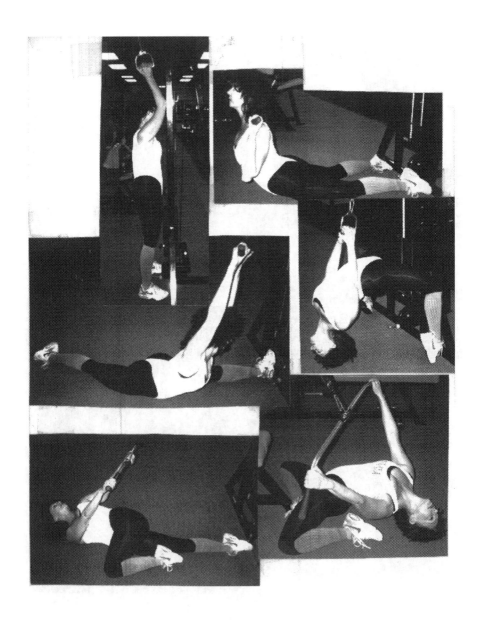

CHAPTER EIGHT
Exploring with Movement

Testing Limits

First, assess the strengths and weaknesses within your body. Then, create movements to explore your motion possibilities, testing the limits of joints, rotations, etc. Always begin slowly with a warm up, making room in the body for the bones to glide through the Breath-Stretch. If during the execution of a movement you feel an unusual strain or your body is far off balance, then relax and allow your body to return to the earth with a soft landing. Creative exercises are inventions requiring more awareness. Proceed gently into this experience. It is the experience of ecstasy and joy in motion that is important, not a competitive skill level.

Explore

You may explore with movement. Explore your abilities. Test your limits. We grow, no matter what our abilities or age, by testing our limits and exploring the unknown. Yes, you may strain your body – so grow little by little. Venture into your own energy world, as only you can, turn perception and sensation into a physical reality. Mind projects energy (*yin*-thought) into body (*yang*-matter). At some point you may over-work or injure an area. Use common sense and rest when necessary. Think about what may be causing the problem. You may need to check movement positioning, check your diet, talk with an enlightened personal trainer or visit a healthcare professional.

Can you get injured? Yes. No easy fix. No fast track. No instantaneous physical evolution. There can be instantaneous mental/ body understanding, but the physical molecules of the body will take time to create the changes that the mind now knows are possible. However, the intuition that you are traveling on the right road will become knowledge of the path as the sensual pathways open. Spirit guides your mind because it understands your experience on this material plane.

The understanding can be immediate, but the development of the body's pathways require time and patience. Let me assure you that the freedom in mind and body that result make the journey worthwhile. The path is not crowded now, but as the spiritual growth of humankind progresses, companions will join you.

Spirit leads the mind out of the common cultural experience into an exciting, motivating thrill deep within, which at once emanates from you and passes through you. Mind becomes steady, resilient, strong, and firm. You find the calm eye of life's storm.

Patience! There is no substitute. Think, feel, act.

At the Gym

The gym may ask you to sign a waiver that states the gym is not responsible for your health and well-being while you are there. Yes, you may hurt yourself. Also, you may be cautioned to not hurt the equipment. Do not bang the weights or pulleys on liftoff or landing.

Someone may approach you and try to make your exercises conform to standard, accepted movements. People are generally afraid of not conforming. Be willing to grant yourself the freedom to experiment and to grant others the freedom to comment on your unique approach.

The following pictures illustrate some weight room exercises.

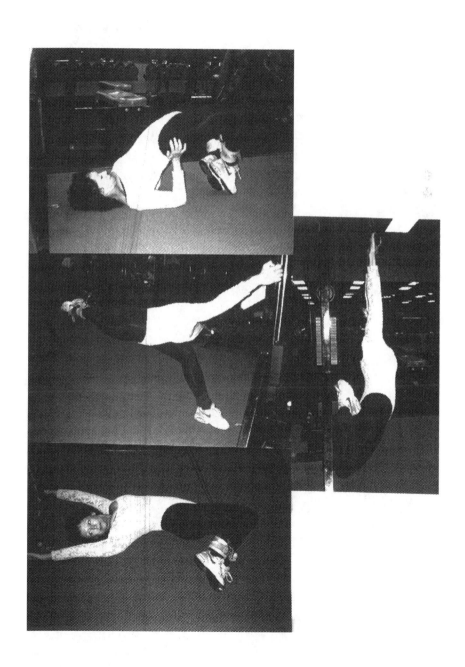

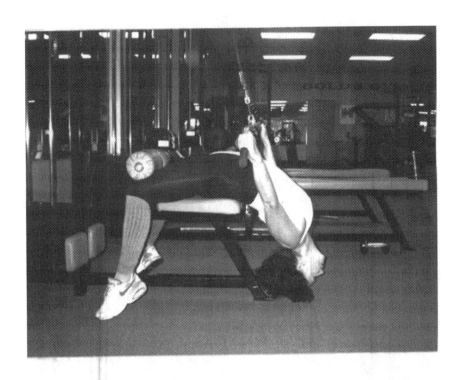

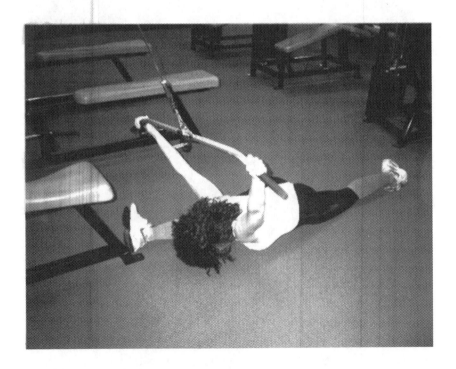

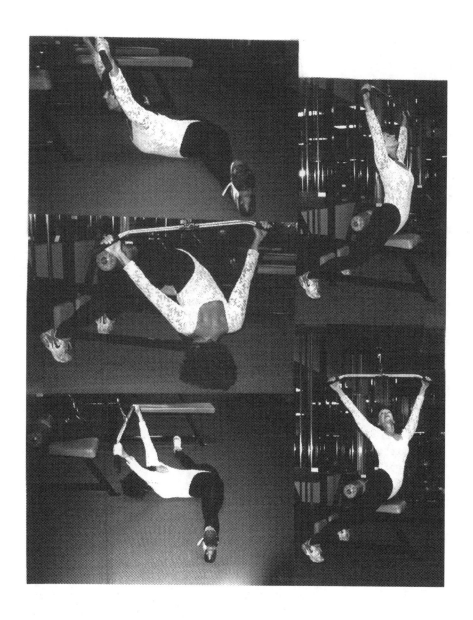

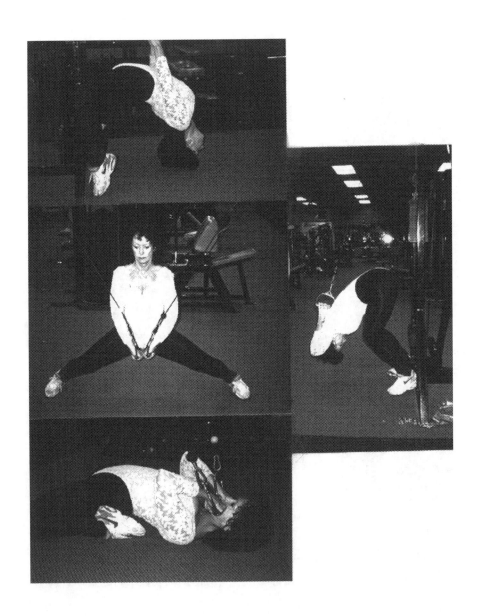

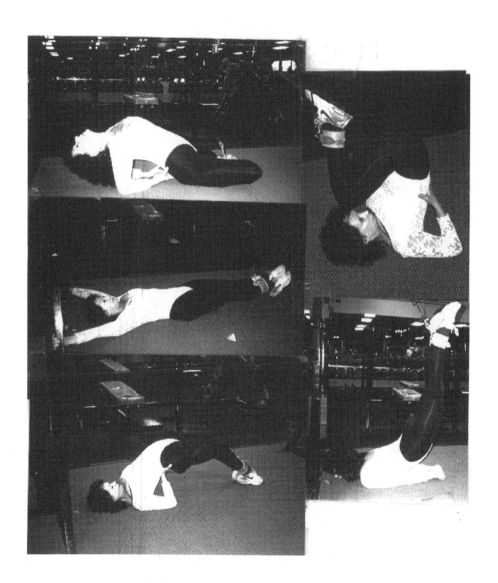

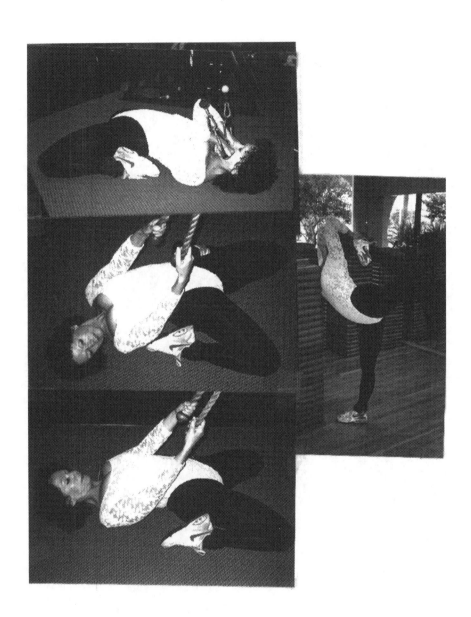

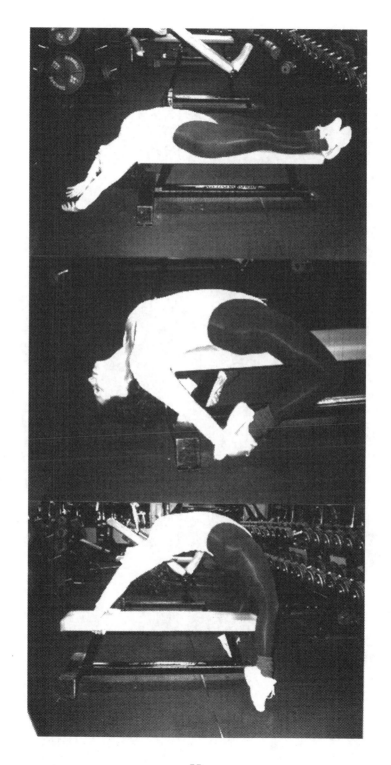

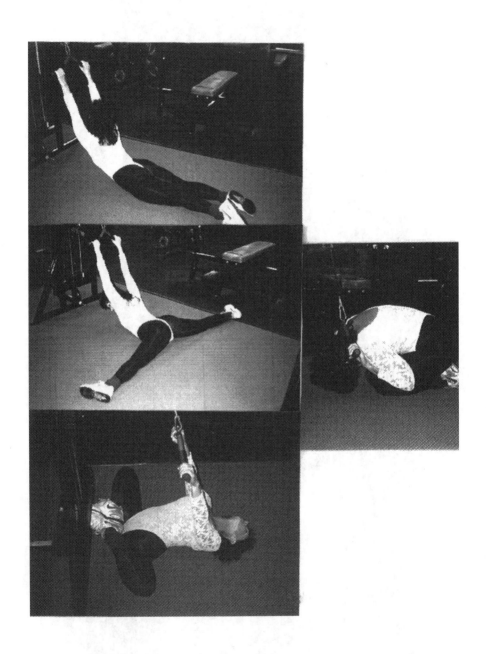

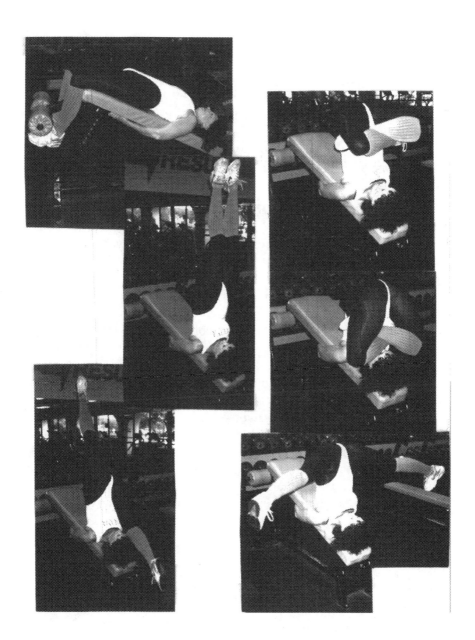

CHAPTER NINE
Water Exercises

Gymnastic Exercises on Land and in Water

The purpose of the exercises is to strengthen and stretch the complete body system. The body systems receive the push or pressure and massage that increases the efficiency of fluid reabsorption and flow. Concentrate on the directional flow of energy with your exercises and build up your own sensual vocabulary to use as a guide along the path of discovery and evolution. Activate the pathways, and the adventure is afoot.

Comparison and Execution

Once the following exercises can be performed with proficiency, combine them into your own creative routine. Before performing an exercise run through the sequence in your mind's eye. Mental practice will ensure a more relaxed and confident performance.

Many of the following exercises on land and in water are based on hatha yoga positions. It is not my intention to describe each movement exactly. Rather, I am giving you the basic activity which you will modify to fit your own performance level.

All the exercises will have an inhalation or exhalation phase to prepare the body for the exercise. Breath will be used in the exercise to focus concentration and be released as the body accomplishes its performance of external motion. In the following exercises if I have not described the preparation breath, then add it. This will give you an impetus to think the sequence though before you move.

Note that an individual's height and flexibility determine his or her **personal range** of movement in the water. So begin slowly! If your pool does not have a gutter, the exercises will need to be adapted to your pool. I suggest a water exercise bar attach to the pool side. ***

Some of the exercises may not be possible. However, it is the thought and inventiveness you apply to the problem that trigger your internal potential. Use your understanding or the breath to help you invent your own exercises. You are now ready to actualize the mind and lead the energy that moves your body.

USE CAUTION

Before practicing any of the exercises in this book, consult your physician concerning your overall health and ability to perform these exercises.

Remember: not all of the exercises are within everyone's skill set. Start slowly and cautiously. **Do less** rather than more. The body will easily perform that which it is prepared to do. It if hurts, stop!

Slight discomfort is to be expected because the physical body changes as the sensations of heat and tingling are produced. However, you must listen to the signals produced by the body to distinguish the changes that are positive from those that indicate too much exertion or strain. Experience is the teacher, and you can evaluate the sensations to determine whether to stop or continue a movement.

When exercising in water, there is the added risk of drowning. Anyone doing water exercises must have someone present and watching at all times – whether the person is a beginner or an expert.

The author is not responsible for any injury to anyone. The ideas, procedures, and suggestions in this booklet are not intended as a substitute for consulting with your physician. All matters regarding your health require medical consultation and supervision.

Before, during and after water gymnastics, stabilizes your body position in the water either by floating on some type of apparatus or anchoring yourself at the gutter or pool side. Perform a few rounds of deep breathing as needed.

* The gutter or bar is the stabilized area on the wall of the pool. Either attached exercise bar or gutter can be used during exercises.

Wear goggles during practice to see pool bottom and sides. Must be in deep enough water not to hit head or legs on the bottom of the pool. Start deeper-at least mid-chest level.

Backward Bending Positions

Cobra (land)
The starting position is facedown with the palms on the ground under your shoulders. You inhale while bending the head and upper back backwards. Breath normally while holding the position; than exhale to return to the starting position.

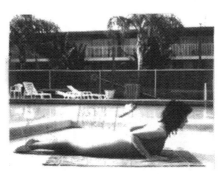

Upper Back Bend (water)
Standing position is with the chest as close as possible to the wall; hold the bar with your hands. As you inhale, bend your head and upper back backward. Breath normally while holding the position; then exhale to return to the starting position.

Variations:
Use your arms by stretching them overhead during the exercise. Perform the exercise, keeping as close to the wall as possible.
After doing upper back bend, continue the exhale forward until you are in a tucked position. Return to the starting position with the body straight to the wall as you inhale.

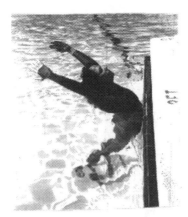

Boat (land)

Lie face down on the ground clasping your hands behind the small of your back. Inhale as you lift your head and upper back with the whole lower body and both legs. Then, exhale to return to the starting position.

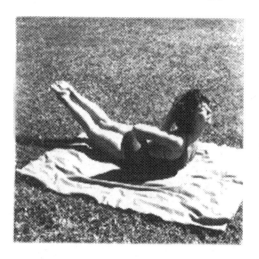

Water Body Wave (water)

To start anchor your toes in the gutter and stretch out face down in the water with your arms straight over your head. Wave or flutter your hands in front of your body to lift your head. Then, take a medium deep breath while arching your hips down. Keep your arms at water level. You exhale in the water as your arch your body and bring your hips to water level.

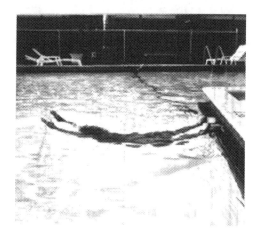

Bow (land)

Starting position is lying face down on the ground. Hold your ankles with your hands and holding your arms straight, inhale as you lift your chest and legs. Come to rest on your abdomen. During the exercise, breath normally while holding the position, and exhale as you come back down to the starting position.

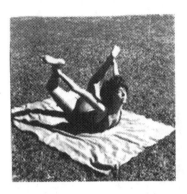

Full Back Bend (water)

Starting position is a layout position face down in the water with the toes anchored on the bar or in gutter. Pull the legs in toward the wall and draw the body toward the wall. To get into the full back bend, exhale while reaching back with one hand to catch the bar. Position the other hand, point the toes toward the pool or keep them flexed. Spread the knees and press forward at the hips. Inhale as you press into the back bend; breathe normally while in the position. To come out of the position, release the hands and float away from the wall.

Variation: Start at the side of the pool. Slide both legs toward the wall behind you and work them up behind you slowly until the toes are in the gutter. Now, position the hand and continue as described above.

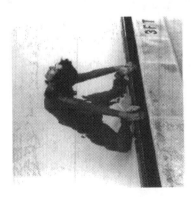

Lion (land)

Starting position is on the ground with the legs either crossed in front of you or tucked under the body Indian style. Inhale deeply; then exhale, forcing the air out the mouth in a gush as you lift the abdomen and curl the buttocks under. To complete the exercise incorporate the face by sticking out the tongue, cross the eyes, and flaring the hands as you exhale.

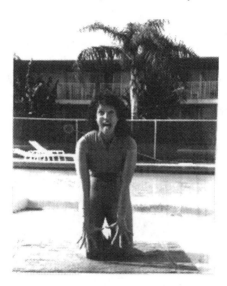

Upper Back Bend On The Wall (water)

Starting position is facing the wall with the legs curled up under the body and the hands holding the gutter. Prepare to move by inhaling as you lift you head and chest backward. To execute the movement, exhale forcefully toward the wall as you stick out your tongue and cross your eyes.

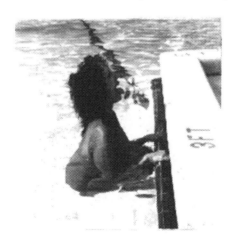

Forward Bending Positions

Half Forward Bend (land)

Starting position is on the ground with one leg extended and the other leg bent inward toward the crotch. Inhale deeply, extending the hands up toward the sky. Exhale, while reaching out to grab ahold of the extended leg with both hands. Hold the position and release tension throughout the body as you hang the head and breath normally. Inhale as you return to the sitting position. Repeat the exercise with the other leg.

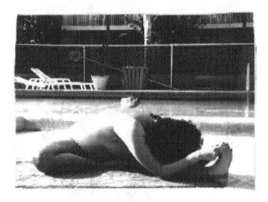

Half Jack-Knife At Wall (water)

Starting position is about three inches from the side of the pool, standing with the pelvis parallel to the wall. Slowly bring one of your feet up the wall to position it out to the side of the body. Continue as described in the above exercise with the heel of the foot in the bar or gutter and the leg as straight as possible. Inhale lifting the arms over the head. Exhale, while reaching out to grab ahold of the extended leg. Relax and breathe normally. To exit the position, inhale while releasing the arms. Repeat the exercise with the other leg.

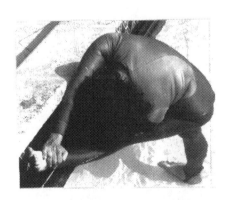

Full Forward Bend (land)

Starting position is seated with legs together and straight out in front of you. Inhale, stretching the arms over head. Exhale, reaching out over the legs and grasping the legs wherever you can reach easily. Hold the position and breath normally. Exit the position by inhaling as you return to a sitting position.

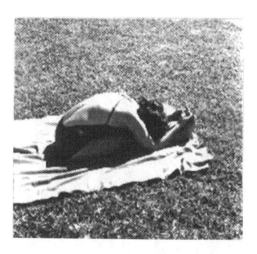

Sustained Jack-Knife (water)

Starting position is in a tuck at the wall of the pool with the toes at the bar or gutter or on the wall behind the bar. Inhale slowly, stretching the legs out if front of you. Exhale, with the legs extended (fingers are grasping the bar to hold the stretch – as you stretch toward the legs). Breath normally as you hold the position. Nose should remain out of the water. Inhale as you return to a crouching position.

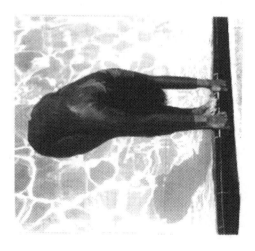

Shoulder Stand (land)

Starting position is lying flat on the back. Exhale, as you lift the legs straight up over the head toward the sky to come to rest on your shoulders. To stabilize yourself, place the hands on the small of the back. Breath normally while holding the position. To exit the position exhale, rolling down on the back and bringing the legs to the ground.

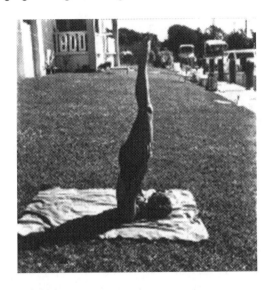

Walled Shoulder Stand (water)

Starting position is "lying" on your back at the water's surface (floating on the back) with the hands behind and overhead holding the bar. Inhale and dig your heels downward, letting the buttocks sink along with the feet as the feet reach the pool's bottom. Chin should remain pressed against the chest. Exhale with feet on the bottom of the pool; feel the increased bend in the neck and shoulder area. Hold the position for a few breaths. Exit position by inhaling to bring body back to the surface as at the beginning. Body should remain straight throughout the exercise.

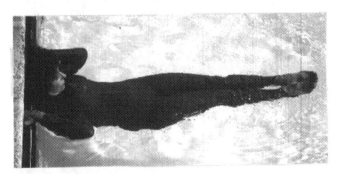

Water Gymnastic Exercises

Side-Stretch Tuck

Side position is with the hands holding the bar and body in a tuck at the wall of the pool. To prepare, exhale; then inhale, bringing both legs up laterally as close as possible to water level. To exit the position, exhale back into a tuck. Repeat the exercise to the other side.

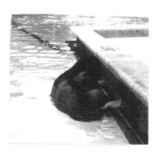 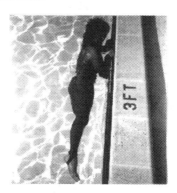

Side Sway

Starting position is with the heels pressing down on the bar or gutter to anchor the body as it floats at the water's surface. Legs should be close together and the arms stretched over the head. To prepare, inhale; then slowly bend the torso to the right as you exhale. Notice that the hips lead the motion. Repeat the motion to the left side.

Variation: Starting position is the same as in the side sway, with the right elbow bent toward the head and the left elbow bent down toward the feet. As the body bends to the right, allow the right elbow sway up toward the head and left elbow to sway down toward the hips. When you reach maximum stretch, change arm positions and repeat the exercise to the other side. (This time, the right elbow sways downward and the left elbow sways upward.)

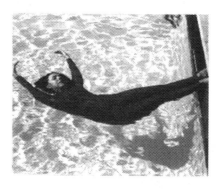

Stag Split with Side Sway

Starting position is face-up with the ankles on the bar or gutter. Begin by inhaling to gain an impetus to move. Bring the arms toward the head while arching the body sideways to the right. Keep the left heel stable in the gutter and exhale as you pull yourself directly toward the pool's side with the left leg, while sliding the right leg along the bar. The full stag split is reached as you complete the exhalation. To exit the position, inhale, allowing the arms to float to the sides of your body and sliding the right leg back along the bar to return to the starting position. Repeat the exercise to the other side.

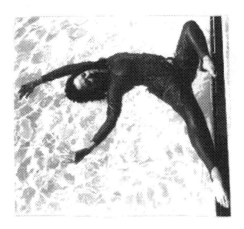

Sit-Ups

Starting position is with the hands holding the bar and the feet at the bar's edge. Slowly slip the lower legs up to rest on the pool's ledge. Slowly slop the lower legs up to rest on the pool's ledge. Inhale to prepare to move; exhale while lifting the head and chest toward the knees. Inhale as you return to the starting position.

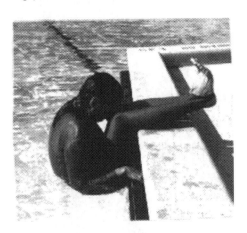

Backward Bend Into A Sit-Up

After completing a sit-up in the previous exercise, return to the starting position and inhale. Bring the body into a Cobra or Upper Back Bend (see above); exhale through the nose as the head enters the water. It is important to exhale continuously through your nose to prevent water from backing up into the nose until you return to the starting position.

Swing and Press

The starting position is face-up, floating with the head almost touching side wall (do not press the head against the wall). The arms are over the head holding the gutter as you focus on the feet. To prepare, inhale; then, exhale and swing the legs to the right while pulling strongly with right arm and right side of the body and right side of the body. Bring the body parallel to the wall. To exit the position inhale, keeping the head at the wall; press gently with the right hand while pulling with the left hand to return the body to the starting position. Breath in a relaxed manner and repeat the exercise to the other side.

Side Split

Starting position is a tuck with the toes curled over the bar or gutter and hands holding the gutter. Inhale as you slowly bring the left leg out in front of you. As the hips turn to the left, keep the heel at the bar's edge; the right leg goes behind with instep riding the edge of bar. Allow the right hand to hold the bar while you bring the left hand over the head. The body should lie back on the surface of the water with the lift arm extended. Relax; allow the body to float and breathe normally. Return to the tuck and repeat the exercise to the other side.

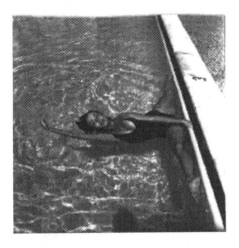

Side-Split Press

Perform the Side Split and leave the right hand on the bar as you exhale. Place the left hand under the left calf and pull the torso toward the leg. While in the position, remain quiet and release all tension. Inhale as you return to the starting position.

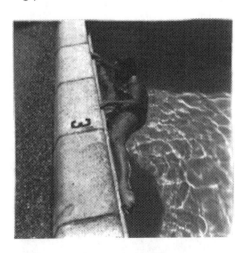

Full Split

Starting position is with the hands holding the bar and the body in a tucked position. Inhale and slowly split both legs with the toes pointing outward and heels riding the edge of the bar. Allow the torso to lie back on the water's surface. Relax while maintaining the position. Exhale as you exit the position and return to the tuck.

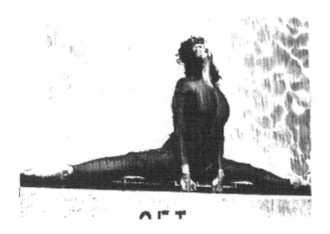

Hip-Joint Split

Starting position is with the body in a tuck and hands holding the bar. Inhale as the knees and legs open. Do not force this opening in any way. Hold the bar with both hands as the buttocks come to rest on the side of the pool. Allow the motion of the water to rock the hip area and loosen it. The breath should remain normal and calm.

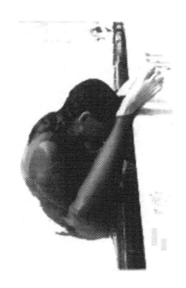

Split Curls

Start in the Full Split position, holding the bar with both hands. Exhale and pull the body up toward the side of the pool using the arms and abdomen. Exhale as you return to the starting position.

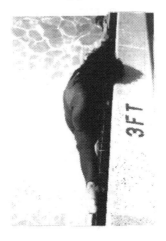

Backward Circulating Flips

Starting position is lying face-up with the hands stretched straight overhead holding the bar. Inhale deeply as you pull with your hands to move the body toward the side of the pool. Because this is a backward somersault, you must begin to exhale through the nose immediately as you duck you head into the water "walk" down the side wall of the pool with the hands. Arch the body into a back bend and continue to "walk" down to and along the bottom of the pool using the hands. Complete the circle by flipping the body so that the head is upward and the feet nearly reach the bottom of the pool. Give a gentle push to the bottom of the pool with the toes to help the body float back up to the starting position. Begin to inhale as soon as your head exits the water and your hands begin reaching for the bar.

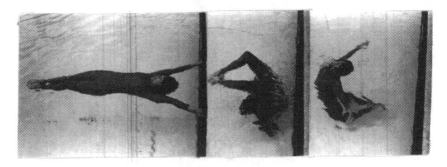

Free Circulating Flips

Starting position is facing the wall in a tuck position with the hands holding the bar and the toes curled over the bar. To prepare inhale; exhale through your nose as the head leads into a back bend. Use a forceful push to the toes on the bar propelling you into the back bend. Keep the toes anchored on the bar as you reach down beside the body toward the bottom of the pool. At maximum back arch, give a push off the gutter with the toes. When your hands reach the bottom of the pool, push on the bottom to direct the hands toward the wall of the pool; "walk" up the wall with the hands. Both hands have reached the bar again, pull the body up out of the water and inhale into another tuck.

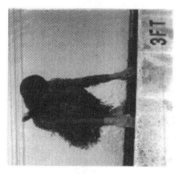 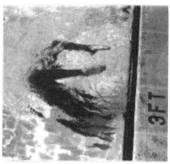

Split Circulating Flips

Starting position is a tuck with hand holding the bar. Inhale as you slide the heels out along the gutter to a full split; the hands should remain extended in front of body holding the bar. Use the head to lead the body backward into a back bend while the arms are extended over the head and down toward the bottom of the pool. As the head enters the water, exhale forcefully through the nose. Draw the legs together and press against the side of the pool to propel the hands toward the bottom of the pool. Touch the bottom of pool with hands before head reaches bottom of the pool (do not allow the head to touch the bottom of the pool). "Walk" along the bottom and up the sides of the pool toward the gutter. When both hands reach the gutter, draw the body back into a tuck. Inhale as the head exits the water.

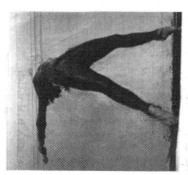 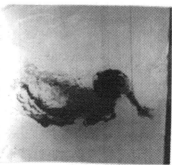

Jack-Knife Flip

Starting position is facing the wall in a tuck with hands holding onto the gutter. Inhale as you straighten the legs and allow the toes to slip off the gutter's edge and point toward the sky. The buttocks move to the wall of the pool and follow the legs over the head. (This is now a somersault in a jack-knife position.) Exhale as the legs move over the head and into a horizontal position keeping the hands on the bar, or as close as possible, while rotating. Return to the starring tuck position and inhale once the head exits the water.

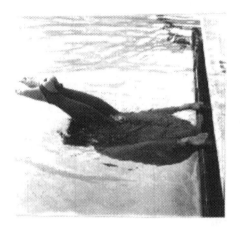

Lotus On The Wall

This movement is a very advanced position.

Assume the lotus position by holding onto the bar with one hand and bring the opposite foot up so that the foot is resting atop the inner thigh of the other leg. Change hands on the bar and slowly work the other leg onto the same position atop the first leg. Hold onto the bar with both hands and rest back onto the surface of the water with the buttocks resting on the bar and perhaps the side of the pool under the bar.

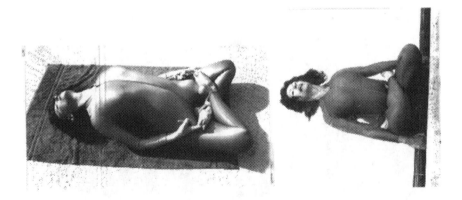

Basic Leg Development Exercises

Leg Swing
Starting position is with the right side of your torso toward the bar and holding the bar with the right hand. Stand on both feet. To begin the motion, exhale swinging the left leg forward toward the surface of the water, and inhale moving the leg backward toward the surface of the water while holding your leg straight. Attempt to keep your body stable as you rest the left arm on the water. After several swings you turn the torso to change legs, and face other direction and repeat the exercise to the other side.

Leg Developer
Starting position is the same as in Leg Swing. You bend the left knee and bring it out to the side to touch the right leg. Now, straighten the left leg forward, keeping the support leg straight, and lower the left leg to the pool's bottom. As you move, feel the hip socket as the thigh swivels. You complete several motions before lifting the leg to the side and straighten. Finally, complete several movements to the back by lifting the knee to the side and straighten the leg to the back. You change sides by tuning the torso to change legs and face the other direction and repeat the exercise to the other side.

Leg Half-Circle
Starting position is the same as the previous exercise, except with the leg stretched straight out in front of you. As you move, keep the leg at the same level in the water. Feel that you are directing a float which supports the leg. Now, inhale circling the leg to the side and back; then exhale, retracing the path to the front of the body. You change sides by turning the torso to change legs and face the other direction. Repeat the exercise to the other side.

Side Leg Kick
Starting position is facing the bar with both hands holding the bar. Inhale, drawing one knee up in front of the body close to the chest. Flex the foot and exhale, kicking out the leg as it straightens to side of the body while attempting to bring the leg perpendicular to the bottom of the pool. Finally, lower the leg to the pool's bottom. Change legs and repeat the exercise several times to the other side.

Side Leg Swing

Starting position is the same as the above exercise. Inhale, lifting the straight leg to the side with the foot flexed; and exhale, lowering the leg to the pool's bottom. Change legs and repeat the exercise several times to the other side.

Figure-8

Starting position is the same as in the Leg Swing with the bent knee in front of the body and foot pointed. Exhale, lifting the knee to follow the top half of a figure-8 pattern. Inhale, digging the knee deeply down into water and passing it behind the other knee and to the side to complete the figure-8 pattern. Change legs and repeat the exercise several times.

Fins

If you are swimming laps across the pool, use regular-sized fins. The leg will have more resistance to overcome. As you move, feel that the origin of the leg is in the center of the body. Kick from the hips with full body motion.

Please, experiment with the exercises and develop your own routine. Increase your range of motion by experimenting with new positions slowly and thoughtfully, applying the Breath-Stretch technique.

CHAPTER TEN
Healing

Body Breath Promotes Healing

Prepare the environment around you so you will not be disturbed, play soft music, assume a comfortable position on the earth or sit in a completely relaxed state.

Begin by watching your thoughts. After a few moments or witnessing the mind, notice that you are the stillness behind the mind's motion. The body will feel extremely heavy (you have given the weight to the earth). This state is similar to the trance-like feeling you have experienced in the twilight state between waking and deep sleep. As you breathe very lightly, you can feel keenly the sweeping sense of breath expansion through the entire body because the physical distractions of gross movement have been eliminated. Also, notice the separation of energy from breath. The vibrating changes that feel like long, gossamer strings are the meridian channels though which energy flows.

In your mind's eye, locate the area of your body that needs healing. Feel the Breath-Stretch in that particular area and concentrate on the electrical flow along the energy pathways from the physical center of the body to the area that needs to be healed. Once this is established, continue to sense the area as you use the power of words (if you are so inclined). Prayer will help you deepen the concentration and build up the will-power to change the material toward which you are directing the energy/charge. If sincere, prayer in any language and any form, will evoke a physical response.

Initially, this state can last anywhere from a few minutes to an hour. You do not lose consciousness and are able to respond to the environment around you if need be. The body goes into "neutral." The power to heal is turned over to the forces of nature that you lead to a specific area.

Your physical body seems to disappear. You feel your bio-electrical system and guide the energy flowing through your body. Observe the natural process as it unfolds. Step back. The natural processes of regeneration and realignment will continue upon their self-determined course.

Wait, feel, experience.

Additional Method of Clearing

Meridian Lines of Energy Motion

On inhalation permit your mind to draw energy up the front of your body from the tips of your fingers and toes through your torso, up to the area of the Third Eye or upper *dan tien*. When you exhale, release the force from the center of your head through the top of your head, down the back of your body, and out the posterior side of your fingers and toes. This method follows the energy lines in the body and allows you to clear any obstructions to the force. Your physical body will be stimulated to heal naturally.

Massage Technique: A Word to the Practitioner

To use Breath-Stretch in massage requires the practitioner to experience it first-hand or at least to have a thorough understanding of the theory. Even if you do not as yet experience Breath-Stretch, the mind, upon understanding the theory, will open up or cue up the sensations and begin their activity.

I will describe two situations that exemplify a technique you can use with your clients. The skilled massage therapist will quickly see that clients respond to the relaxation experienced. This will enable the therapist to work more deeply on difficult therapeutic applications. Most important, explain to the client the theory behind Breath-Stretch. Client participation is of utmost importance. Tell the client that he or she is expanding and releasing from within the body. Explain that the breath acts like a hand producing waves of pressure and release deep within the body, and that as you exhale, you send energy through painful areas to dissolve the problem.

Therapeutic Applications

Static Stretches

In this technique the therapist positions the body area which is constricted or in trauma in a passive stretch position. For example, have your patient lie on his or her back with one knee drawn up toward the chest while you press the knee toward the chest. Ask the client to breath from the abdomen, expanding down through the lower back, buttocks, into the leg, and all the way down to and through the toes. Tell him or her to feel the fluids press against the skin on inhalation. Feel the fluids release and send energy down the leg and through the tight areas to be released on exhalation. Press the knee lightly further into the stretch. Maintain the position while the client takes the next Breath-Stretch inhalation. Continue for a number of breaths and have the client come out of the stretch while inhaling.

Lumps of Contracted Tissue

Therapist must locate the area of contraction or trauma. Press the side of the problem area nearest the center of the patient's body. Tell the patient to feel his or her breath reach up toward the tissue, producing increased pressure. The patient should be directed to feel the pressure decrease and the problem area dissolve on exhalation. Do not produce pain so that the client wishes to withdraw. Discomfort, however, is acceptable. Tell the client to feel that his or she is drawing the breath toward the problem area as the internal pressure increases on inhalation, engulfing the pain. On exhalation the client should disperse the pain into space as energy passes through the tissue and the internal pressure decreases.

The experienced, licensed massage professional will be able to speak to a client creatively and master this technique after experiencing the Breath-Stretch technique first-hand. This booklet can enlighten the pathway within you. Creative exploration with your clients will carry you both forward toward your individual destinations.

APPENDIX
Recap of Breath-Stretch's Two
Movement Phases: *Yin/Yang* Cycle

INHALE = *Yin* Cycle

Characteristics:

- Buildup of energy
- Contraction of diaphragm: the lymph system backs up
- Can be accompanied by muscle-release pattern exercise such as return to the norm or the negative energy motion in weight training (see Chapter 7)

EXHALE = *Yang* Cycle

Characteristics:

- Sending of force
- Forced expulsion and release of muscular tension as diaphragm relaxes; the lymph system moves forward
- Can be accomplished by muscle-force pattern in physical exercise such as the active phase (a strike in martial arts) or the positive energy motion in weight training

Other Names for Life Force or Energy

China	*chi* or *qu*
Japan	*ki*
India	*prana*
Russia	bioplasmic energy
Western World	bioelectricity
Wilhelm Reich	orgone energy
Old Testament	breath of life

BIBLIOGRAPHY

Chia, Mantak. *Iron Shirt Chi Kung I*. Huntington, N.Y.: Healing Tao Books, 1986.

Friedman, Norman. *Bridging Science and Spirit*. St. Louis: Living Lake Books, 1994.

Gerber, Robert. *Vibrational Medicine*. Santa Fe: Bear & Company, 1988.

Goswami, Shyan Sundar. *Hatha-Yoga*. London: L. N. Fowler & Co, 1963.

Man-ching, Cheng. *Tai Chi Chuan*. Taiwan: China Engraving and Printing Works, 1963.

Yang, Jwing-Ming. *Muscle/Tendon Changing and Marrow/Brain Washing Chi Kung*. Jamaica Plain, Mass: Yang's Martial Arts Association, 1989.

GLOSSARY

Bio-environment: The environment in which a living organism exists.

Buddhism: An ancient Indian religion that advocates meditation for spiritual and physical development.

Chakra: An energy center in the body. Chakras process subtle energy and convert it into chemical, hormonal and cellular changes in the body.

Chi (or Qi): Chinese term for the vital life-energy force, which includes heat, light and electromagnetic energy. *Chi* is a subtle nutritive energy that circulates through the acupuncture meridian.

Dan Tien: The three places in the body where *chi* is stored. They are: the upper *dan tien* (located between the eyebrows): the middle *dan tien* (at the solar plexus); and the lower *dan tien* (a few inches below the navel).

Diaphragm: The main muscle involved in the breathing process, located between the chest and abdominal cavities.

Ki: Internal energy; the Japanese term for the subtle nutritive energy that flow through the acupuncture meridians.

Lymph: Specialized fluid formed in the tissue spaces that return excess fluid and protein molecules to the blood.

Lymphatic System: A system that plays a critical role in the functioning or the immune system, moves fluids and large molecules from the tissue spaces, and fat-related nutrients from the digestive system to the blood.

Prana: Indian term for the universal vital force that is found in the sun, the air and the earth, and which keeps the body alive and healthy: yogic term for a subtle nutritive energy thought to be taken in during breathing. It is referred to in Ayurvedic medicine.

Taoism: An ancient religion of China. The "natural" way of everything.

Vital Force: That which defines life; known as *chi/qi, ki* and *prana*.

Yang: In Chinese philosophy the active, positive, masculine polarity.

Yin: In Chinese philosophy the passive, negative, feminine polarity.

Yoga: Method of physical, mental and spiritual development. The work is derived from the Sanskrit word meaning "union".

ABOUT THE AUTHOR

Dr. Wendy Gross received her Doctorate in Healthcare Leadership from Nova University; degree of Master of Arts from Columbia University, Teachers College; degree of Master of Science from Barry University; and degree of Bachelor of Arts from University of Florida. She has been a yoga teacher for 45 years and licensed massage therapist for 21 years with licenses in Arizona, Nevada, and Florida. Her last academic position was Department Head Massage Specialist, College of Southern Nevada in Las Vegas, NV. Currently, she is on-call at Jupiter Medical Center, Lighthouse Detox Center for massage and yoga.

During her philosophy classes in college Dr. Gross discovered that yoga linked the mind and body in a sensation experience. This understanding compelled her to explore the classical and innovative movement styles of both Eastern and Western cultures.

Breath-Stretch technique is the foundation of the energy experience expressed on land and water.

Energy follows the breath and the mind directs the attention of consciousness toward the desired experience.

Contact Information email: wlgross@earthlink.net
Topics of Interest:
To Have Group or Individual Seminars on Land or Water Program – contact
    Dr. Gross for scheduling, etc.
Ordering Exercise Bar for Water Program – contact Dr. Gross for equipment
    suggestions
Available: Sensational Water Fitness/Yoga: Demonstration of Water
    Exercises
    Color Video - 15 minute
    Email for details

Printed in the United States
By Bookmasters